The International Behavioural and Social Sciences Library

DATE DUE

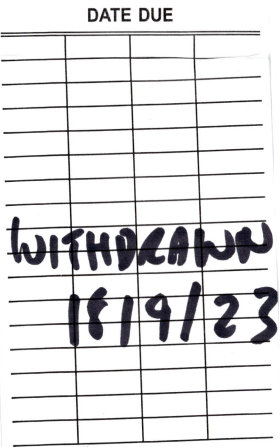

The International Behavioural and Social Sciences Library

PSYCHIATRY
In 5 Volumes

PSYCHIATRY IN A CHANGING SOCIETY

EDITED BY S H FOULKES
AND G STEWART PRINCE

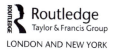

Routledge
Taylor & Francis Group

LONDON AND NEW YORK

First published in 1969 by
Tavistock Publications Limited

Reprinted in 2001 by
Routledge
2 Park Square, Milton Park, Abingdon, Oxon, OX14 4RN
Simultaneously published in the USA and Canada by Routledge
711 Third Avenue, New York, NY 10017

Transferred to Digital Printing 2007

First issued in paperback 2013

Routledge is an imprint of the Taylor & Francis Group, an informa business

The publishers have made every effort to contact authors/copyright holders
of the works reprinted in the *International Behavioural and Social Sciences
Library*. This has not been possible in every case, however, and we would
welcome correspondence from those individuals/companies we have been
unable to trace.

These reprints are taken from original copies of each book. In many cases
the condition of these originals is not perfect. The publisher has gone to
great lengths to ensure the quality of these reprints, but wishes to point
out that certain characteristics of the original copies will, of necessity, be
apparent in reprints thereof.

British Library Cataloguing in Publication Data
A CIP catalogue record for this book
is available from the British Library

Psychiatry in a Changing Society

ISBN 978-0-415-26475-4 (hbk)
ISBN 978-0-415-86905-8 (pbk)

Psychiatry in a Changing Society

Edited by
S. H. FOULKES and
G. STEWART PRINCE

TAVISTOCK PUBLICATIONS
London . New York . Sydney . Toronto . Wellington

First published in 1969
by Tavistock Publications Limited
2 Park Square, Milton Park, Abingdon, Oxon, OX14 4RN
Editorial matter © S. H. Foulkes and G. S. Prince
in 11 pt Garamond 1 pt leaded

ISBN 422 71930 7

Distributed in the USA
by Barnes & Noble, Inc.

Contents

Acknowledgements

'Psychosis and Social Change among the Tallensi of Northern Ghana' by Professor Meyer Fortes and Dr Doris Y. Mayer was first published in *Cahiers d'Études Africaines* (EPHE, VI, Sorbonne), Vol. 6 (1), No. 21, 1966, and is republished here, with some amendments, by permission of the Editor.

'Managers, Men, and the Art of Listening' by Professor R. W. Revans is reprinted from *New Society*, 4 February 1965, pp. 13-15, with the Editor's permission.

A fuller version of 'Psychology and the Ideology of Progress' by Professor Paul Halmos forms part of his book *The Faith of the Counsellors*, published by Constable, London, in 1965, and by Schocken, New York, in 1966.

The passage from 'Typical Medical Students' by Dr H. J. Walton is reprinted from the *British Medical Journal*, 1964, Vol. 2, pp. 744-8, by permission of the Author, Editor, and Publishers.

Excerpts from 'Sickness and the Social Compact' by Dr Alan Parkin are reprinted from the *Canadian Psychiatric Association Journal*, 1964, Vol. 9, No. 4, by permission of the Author and Editor.

In the chapter entitled 'The Issue', Dr S. H. Foulkes has drawn on his earlier paper 'Illness as a Social Process', which was published in *Psychotherapy and Psychosomatics*, 1966, Vol. 14.

Introductory

G. STEWART PRINCE and S. H. FOULKES

The papers appearing in this volume were all presented to the Psychotherapy and Social Psychiatry Section of the Royal Medico-Psychological Association in 1965 and one of us (S.H.F.) was Chairman of the Section. We believe that they raise issues of interest and importance which cannot be confined within the relatively narrow frontiers of a scientific psychiatric group. It is, after all, one of the most convincing evidences of change within our society that attitudes towards mental illness, mental health, and mental development have altered dramatically in the last few decades. The popularity, for instance, of 'Lifeline', a programme devoted to psychiatric topics, was such that it was seen on television by eight million people at a time, and a number of well-informed, well-written popular books on psychiatric subjects have been best-sellers. This particular evidence of recent change within our society can, however, more soberly be studied by a brief review of the history of formal psychiatry in Britain.

In 1841 the Royal Medico-Psychological Association was set up in London with the prime aim of promoting the scientific study of mental illness by practitioners of medicine. As the Association expanded and knowledge slowly increased, various subcommittees were formed to represent special interests, and eventually some of these were converted into Sections of the Association.

In 1948 the Council of the Association recommended to the Social Psychiatry Section that it enlarge its scope to include psychotherapy, and it was transformed in 1949 into the Psychotherapy and Social Psychiatry Section, one of the biggest in the Association, and today boasting well over a thousand members.

The inaugural meeting of the new Section was held in April 1949, and short addresses were given by senior psychotherapists on the role of psychotherapy within psychiatry. From then on, the

scientific meetings of the Section were increasingly concerned
with psychotherapeutic topics as well as with the social aspects of
psychiatry. Psychoanalysts and others identified with psychotherapy began to attend the meetings in increasing numbers and
to undertake committee work and to hold office. By 1953 the
Section Committee found it necessary seriously to review the role
of the Section. It was concluded that the most important task for
the next few years was the spreading of psychotherapy in Britain,
and particularly the teaching of psychotherapeutic techniques,
but the difficulties of achieving this aim, especially for psychiatrists in outlying mental hospitals and in the provinces, were
clearly recognized. A certain unease about the standing of the
Section and its relation to the broad stream of British psychiatry
made itself felt. It was therefore suggested that the Committee
should co-opt members representing the British Psycho-Analytical
Society, the Society of Analytical Psychology, and the Medical
Section of the British Psychological Society, to further the basic
aim and to improve liaison with these Societies.

A period of energetic discussion and planning followed,
invigorating to the administration of the Section and the membership, but it would be fair to comment that the aim of spreading
psychotherapy was never fully realized. It is true today that
psychotherapy is by no means evenly spread over Britain.

By 1956 the Section had become strong enough to advocate
monthly meetings, and a foretaste of things to come was given
by a series of papers under the general heading of 'The mental
hospital as a therapeutic community'. These papers might have
realigned the psychotherapists with their colleagues concerned
with other aspects of psychiatry, but in the event they failed to do
so. In general, the Section increased its interest in psychotherapeutic subjects and the influence of social psychiatry appeared to
wane, although by no means to disappear. By 1957 psychotherapeutic specialism had reached the point at which a large meeting
listened to Miss Anna Freud discussing problems arising in connection with the ending of treatment in child analysis—a notable
event, but a far cry from the prime aim of the Section in 1953.

The social psychiatry interest was mainly symbolized by the
provision of visits to mental hospitals and specialized treatment
units, and by the presentation of papers by senior mental nurses –
a welcome innovation. The problem of providing widespread

training in psychotherapy continued to defy solution in spite of much labour and discussion.

By December 1958 the Section had got round to studying its problems scientifically, and this phase was symbolized by a meeting at which a research psychiatrist described an investigation of a group of seventy-eight psychiatrists designed to measure sympathy with analytic or organic attitudes. These were found to be negatively related, although not diametrically opposed. An analyst countered with a statement on the analytical attitude.

In March 1959 the position was surveyed from the vantage-point of the Chair of Psychiatry at the Maudsley Hospital. The message for the future offered by Sir Aubrey Lewis was a plea for the greater recognition by psychiatrists of the social sciences. This book may be a tribute to his wisdom. By December of that year a reconciling concept seemed to be promised in a paper entitled 'Psychopathology of social processes'. However, splitting rather than reconciling forces were in the ascendant. Time and study were adding prestige to the concept of social psychiatry, and the slowly increasing number of research posts for senior psychiatrists gave the epidemiology of psychiatry a growing influence.

Finally, in 1961, a member of the Section Committee resigned on the ground that the Section was not concerning itself with his conception of social psychiatry but rather with psychotherapy. Both in the Committee and in Section meetings much time was devoted to discussion, argument, scientific papers, and symposia, in an effort to clarify definitions. 'What is psychotherapy?' 'What is social psychiatry?' And 'What is the relation between the two?' No conclusive answers emerged, although much that was thought-provoking was said. The Committee seemed to split into segregationist and unionist camps. Dr Foulkes and I, the editors of this volume, took up an integrationist position and looked outside psychiatry to speakers from other disciplines who might illustrate our belief that the key to the conflict lies in the fact that psychiatry is evolving rapidly in an even more rapidly changing society.

In the face of such a situation in a group there are a number of alternative ways of dealing with the matter. The conflict can be ignored or even denied, or the situation can be accepted and an attempt made to manipulate it. Alternatively, it can be taken up as the main and most urgent theme for the attention of the group. In my position as Chairman Elect to the Section, I (S.H.F.), with my group-analytic orientation, decided for this last course.

My experience had made me familiar with this kind of split in many situations. It occurs characteristically when a group is confronted with deep-going issues of principle. I had observed this in therapeutic groups as well as in seminar groups of trainee psychiatrists. Having observed it, I found descriptions of the same type of split arising under similar conditions (Foulkes, 1964, pp. 249–50, 252–4; Hunter, unpublished). This particular split occurs typically between those members of a group who wish to be more personally involved and who are ready to accept change – including change in their own person – and those members who resist change. There was every reason to assume that the issue facing the present group of psychiatrists was of this nature. Those who do not wish to be exposed to change would like to keep away from dynamic interventions such as psychotherapy, psychoanalysis, or group analysis. They are therefore in favour of 'scientific investigation', which to them means a stable situation, free of all intervention. The same type of difference in attitude may be seen throughout psychiatry but equally well throughout all other fields of human endeavour and investigation at the present time.

The reason why we find these same signs of disturbance in all spheres lies ultimately, in my opinion, in the rapid change of Western society, including our own, with which we cannot keep pace and which emphasizes the areas of particular maladjustment and stress. The behaviour that we are just now discussing corresponds to a very widespread method of defence against openly facing true sources of conflict. The result is a polarization. The disturbance becomes precipitated in one faction of the community who, according to their inclination, may contrive to be psychotics, neurotics, delinquents, bearers of apparent or real physical diseases, or just more and more common or garden miserable persons. The others can then locate the trouble in them and say that they want to study it quantitatively and qualitatively in order to establish its 'causes' and take appropriate precautions. What is thus put out of sight is that the whole trouble in all its different manifestations is a symptom and result of a disturbance in the balance of society and community life.

For our purposes, in the field of psychiatry itself, who turns to which side of the conflict may be determined in the first place by basic personality attributes. My own impression is that we are confronted with two types of person: those who like to isolate and departmentalize and those who wish to synthesize and integrate. Even these deeper personality factors can and should be understood also in terms of a sociological analysis of these attitudes.

H. J. Walton (1964) has found a similar typology among medical students. I quote his summary of his article 'Typical medical students':

'In a class of 102 graduating medical students, four composite doctors have been defined by a statistical technique, "delegate analysis", based on sixty-six attitudinal and criterion measures. Two of the doctors representing the class are organically oriented, while two are interested in non-organic illness and the psychological and social aspects of patients.

The first organically oriented doctor, although confining his medical interest to a narrowly physical approach, was labelled "adequate"; he has a positive or neutral relationship to patients as people, and is relaxed in his attitude towards them. The second organically oriented doctor was termed "limited"; he is characterized by rancour towards all patients who do not have serious organic illness to which he confines his anxious and irritable attention. The two other representatives were both interested in social and emotional aspects of illness. The third composite graduate is "research-oriented"; he has scientific attitudes and an interest in technical procedures. The last graduate is "patient-centred"; he considered that medical students should see patients from the start of their training. He is characterized by his interest in the social and psychological problems of patients and is a potential psychiatrist.'

A valuable contribution for our present purpose is a paper by Alan Parkin, read at the Annual Meeting of the Canadian Psychiatric Association in 1963, under the title 'Sickness and the social compact'. I give some excerpts here because they have immediate importance for us:

'The result is . . . that patients of a particular social class find themselves therapeutically engaged with psychiatrists of a particular social and personal ideology. There is thus formed a *social compact* between patient and doctor which not only may determine the outcome of the treatment process but also may define the nature of the illness itself. There was a direct relation between social class and the prevalent rates for the depressive reactions, the obsessive compulsive reactions, and the character neuroses. The rates of the latter were six times higher in the upper social classes than in the lower. The sole exception amongst the neuroses was hysteria, for which the prevalent rates were markedly higher in the lower social classes. . . . Thus the culture of the upper social class predisposed to the development of *symptoms* expressive of *psychological* conflict while that of the lower social class predisposed to the development of *behaviour* expressive of *social* conflict.'

As to the psychiatrists themselves, Parkin, following Hollingshead and Redlich's famous study (1958), discerns the 'directive organic group' and the 'analytic psychologic group':

'The ideology of the first group is closer to that of the medical profession as a whole. These psychiatrists carry out physical and neurological examinations on their patients; they treat them by various physical methods such as shock, surgery and drugs; their psychotherapy is of the nature of direction, manipulation, suggestion, advice, reassurance and persuasion; they read the general medical journals and belong to the general medical societies; their social affiliations are with the general medical profession; and they wear white coats in their practices. . . . They attribute their becoming psychiatrists to the needs of the patients in this field and to the opportunities to help them. They tend to deny the existence of social classes or are embarrassed by the fact. In one study 42 per cent of this group had moved up one or more social classes from the position occupied by their fathers.

The second group of analytical psychiatrists and psychoanalysts share a professional and personal ideology different from that of the medical profession as a whole. They eschew the carrying out of physical and neurological examinations and refer their patients to colleagues for these procedures; they forgo the various physical methods of treatment; their psychotherapy is of the nature of analysing the patient's behaviour, feelings and thoughts in terms of deeper motives; they read psychoanalytic journals and belong to psychotherapeutic societies; their social affiliations are with other than the general medical group; and they wear business suits in their practices.... They attribute their becoming psychiatrists to their own child-hood problems and their attempts to solve them. They are interested in the fact of social gratification and have opinions concerning its determinants. In the same study 75 per cent of this group had moved up one or more social classes from the position occupied by their fathers.

There is a strong suggestion here of the social determination of the professional ideology of doctors as a whole, which is in need of further clarification. It may be significant that this clarification has been achieved to a greater extent among the psychiatric group.'

With regard to the concept of social compact, Parkin leans or builds upon work by Talcott Parsons:

'Thus every doctor-patient relationship may be regarded as a *social compact*, the implicit terms of which are accepted by each as binding upon himself. The terms of expectation and obliga-tion of the *traditional* medical ideology so encumber this social compact when it is joined for psychiatric purposes that it must inevitably fail by making it either easier to be ill or impossible to be well. The only possible way of proceeding is to open the compact itself for investigation and its terms for negotiation. This procedure, at the same time, brings one to grips with the terms of the illness itself.'

This excursion gives perhaps a foretaste of social psychiatry as I should like to see it understood.

For all these reasons I thought it a good idea to dramatize the conflict within the Section by making it the basis of discussion for a whole year's programme or maybe even for several years. The actual problem did not appear to be a very important one. There seems to be no doubt that a body like the Royal Medico-Psycho-logical Association will have ample need and scope for a Section on psychotherapy as well as for a more research-oriented Section including social psychiatry, and Dr Hare has stated the case for separation very clearly.

It is not irrelevant to mention that, at this stage of the established organization of psychiatry, the present Section serving social psychiatry and psychotherapy is not on the main road of interest of psychiatrists. When its meetings coincide with the quarterly sessions of the whole RMPA they are well visited; otherwise attendance is poor except when a special subject or a known speaker exerts a particular attraction. Psychiatrists come to this Section mainly in the hope of picking up some useful practical or theoretical help in psychotherapy, in which their training is often sadly inadequate.

Another reason why we have decided to publish the proceedings of the year in this volume is in order to make them available now and in the future to those who are interested.

To me it seems that there is a need for a new orientation in social psychiatry as well as in psychotherapy; that psychiatry itself will be subjected to change in view of changing social and cultural conditions, with the result that the whole of psychiatry will have to become more conscious of social and cultural factors. In this sense the whole of psychiatry is social psychiatry as well.

This Section will be needed, in my opinion, to cultivate a new dimension of psychiatry as well as of psychotherapy, and also an integration with many other disciplines, medical and non-medical. It would not greatly matter what such a section was called, but either Social Psychiatry or Cultural Psychiatry would seem to be a suitable title. In my address from the Chair I suggested that, if the present Section remained united, a mere change of emphasis would be useful, namely, Section for Social Psychiatry and Psychotherapy.

The main idea behind the year's programme was to demonstrate that these problems exist and that different disciplines encounter the same problems within their own provinces although they are largely ignorant of each other; that this is not accidental; that the problems are psychiatric and affect the community as a whole. Within the year we could not do more than marshal evidence for these views; to make the evidence available for further discussion and analysis is the primary object of the present book.

It will be clear, too, why the speakers, now contributors to this volume, are not predominantly psychiatrists. Their work is in education, anthropology, sociology, social psychiatry, and industry. The value of their testimony is enhanced by the fact that it is drawn from a wide variety of fields.

In the first part of the book, this introduction and the first two chapters, the issue is stated; Part II comprises contributions that relate to particular fields; those that have adopted a more theoretical approach constitute Part III; conclusions are presented in Part IV.

The material presented in Parts II and III not only reveals problems but indicates a variety of approaches to their study and solution. The issues explored are obviously of particular importance for all psychiatrists, psychoanalysts, and psychotherapists. They are, however, of no less consequence for all anthropologists, sociologists, teachers, politicians, artists, industrialists, and others.

We hope that this symposium will be successful in bringing this work to the knowledge of at least a representative section of the community.

The problem displayed in the Psychotherapy and Social Psychiatry Section is a symptom and sign of a deep-seated issue in psychiatry in general as well as in the society of which psychiatry is a part. Indeed, it appears to be the most urgent issue that psychiatry as a whole faces today. Its solution is a precondition if action is to be fruitful. The testimony of speakers from fields far separated from each other confirms the universality of psychiatric problems in the community and the need for psychiatrists to become aware of these problems; to diagnose them and to analyse them so as to be able to advise on and participate in appropriate treatment. If the psychiatrist is to accomplish this task he must have an integrated view over the entire field now split up into so many departments. He will then understand why these problems are so closely related in their character and he will be able to take up his legitimate place in social therapy and social research.

REFERENCES

FOULKES, S. H. (1964). *Therapeutic group analysis*. London: Allen & Unwin.
HOLLINGSHEAD, A. B. & REDLICH, F. C. (1958). *Social class and mental illness: a community study*. New York: Wiley.

B

HUNTER, R. C. A. (Unpublished). Teach or treat. (Referred to in Foulkes, 1964.)

PARKIN, A. (1964). Sickness and the social compact. *Canadian psychiat. Assoc. J.* **9**, 4.

WALTON, H. J. (1964). Typical medical students. *Br. med. J.* (ii), 744–8.

Part I: Two Opposed Views of Social Psychiatry

1 The Relation between Social Psychiatry and Psychotherapy

E. H. HARE

Social psychiatry includes a diversity of interests and activities, and it has become a question whether all these can be adequately catered for in one Section of the Royal Medico-Psychological Association, a Section that also caters for the multifarious and vigorous appetites of psychotherapy. My purpose is first of all to examine the evolution of the term 'social psychiatry', and to contrast the ways in which it has been used by different authorities. I shall then put forward the view that the term social psychiatry can be seen to comprise three more or less distinct and self-contained subjects. I shall examine the relation of these subjects to psychotherapy and, finally, offer the opinion that one of the subjects would find a better soil for its development if it left the cover of social psychiatry and the arena of psychotherapy.

CONNOTATION OF TERMS

In order to consider the relation between social psychiatry and psychotherapy, one must first determine what is meant by these two terms. And here, at once, is a great difficulty. Not only does the term social psychiatry mean different things to different people, but the various things of which it is thought to be made up are constantly changing in shape and size and consistency. Aristotle held that, among the several different meanings a word may have, the particular meaning intended on any occasion can be deduced from the context in which it is used. This is all very well for a word whose different meanings are clearly recognized, so that all the hearer or reader has to do is to decide which of its various usages is intended. But the trouble with a new and rapidly evolving term is that people disagree on what the various possible meanings are, so that to understand it on any occasion

one needs to know not only its verbal context but also the prefer-
ences and prejudices of the person who is using it – in rather the
same way as a candidate, considering what to say at a viva voce
examination, may pay as much attention to the known eccentricities of his examiner as to the question asked. For the real meaning
of such terms, a modern analogy might be the position of an
electron which, we are told, cannot be located in the ordinary
sense of being either here or there, but can only be represented
by a fog of probability. Our task, to determine the relation of
two fogs of probability, is not an easy one.

PSYCHOTHERAPY

I shall make the task easier by a rather cavalier treatment of the
term 'psychotherapy'. I can do this because it is a word that has
been in common use for many decades, and the image that it
presents to the mind has had time to solidify from its primal
chaos. True, a recent reviewer said that the term psychotherapy
has been used to describe activities which may range all the way
from colouring a pill to a formal Freudian analysis lasting half
a lifetime. Yet I think there would be general agreement, first,
that psychotherapy is a form of *therapy*, that is to say, it is an
activity essentially concerned with the treatment of patients; and,
second, that it is closely connected with theories of psychodynamics and psychopathology.

SOCIAL MEDICINE

We can now approach the general subject of social psychiatry.
One way of doing this is to consider it as a logical development
of social medicine. I have not looked closely into the origin of
the term 'social medicine',[1] but it first became widely used in
Britain during the early 1940s when it was popularized by the
late Professor John Ryle. Ryle was particularly interested in
peptic ulcer and he recognized that, though laboratory and
clinical studies could determine the pathological processes and the
best ways of treatment, yet they could not indicate the prevalence
of peptic ulcer in the community, or whether the prevalence was
increasing or decreasing, or why or to what extent this prevalence
varied in different groups of people. In other words, clinical and

[1] The historical development of the concept of social medicine may be
examined in Sand (1948, 1952), Galdston (1954), and Anderson (1965).

laboratory studies could not elucidate the social factors in disease. From this, he was led to the view that medical teaching and research ought to become increasingly concerned with these social factors, and that the nose of orthodox medicine had been too close to the hospital bed and the laboratory bench to be sufficiently aware of the physical and psychological miasmata from the factory and the home.

In 1942, at Oxford, Ryle became the holder of the first Chair of Social Medicine in Britain, and in 1947 he gave the following definition of social medicine. It embraces, he said, 'on the one hand, the whole of the activities of public health administration and of the remedial and allied social services, and, on the other, the special disciplines necessary for the advancement of knowledge relating to sickness and health in the community' (Ryle, 1948). Notice there are three parts to this definition, parts which we shall meet again, with more or less emphasis, in the definitions of social psychiatry. The three parts are: public health administration; remedial and allied social services; and disciplines for the advancement of knowledge. In other words: administration, therapy, and research. The research aspects of social medicine he called 'social pathology', because he held there was a precise analogy between the social factors in disease, as studied by social medicine, and the anatomical and physiological factors, as studied by clinical medicine; and in this sense he refers to the study of death-rates and correlated factors as 'the social post-mortem examination'.

Ryle had a *penchant* for new terms. 'Hygiology' was the study of health and its causes, but it was a term that seems to have been still-born, perhaps because of the difficulty of defining health in other than negative terms. Ryle had a flair for public relations as well as for new terms, and I sometimes wonder how far his choice of the term social medicine was determined by its euphony – contrast the awkward word epidemiology and its tongue-twisting derivations – and how far by the good public image it had in the early 'forties. At that time there was much planning for the coming postwar era; Lord Beveridge's proposals for social security were being widely acclaimed; and with the advent of the socialist government to power in 1945, the seal of approval for the adjective in Britain was confirmed. This is not fanciful, for it is commonly agreed that one reason why the terms social medicine and social psychiatry have made less headway in the United States than in Britain is the bad image with the American public, and particularly with the medical profession, of any term homophonous with 'socialism'.

We might pause here for a moment to consider whether the fate of the term social medicine gives us any clue as to the prognosis of the term social psychiatry. On the one hand, we can reflect that social medicine is not a term, or even a subject, that has found much favour in those foci of tradition, the medical schools; and I have heard an eminent teacher, reflecting on the Department of Social Medicine at Oxford, shake his head sadly and refer to 'poor Ryle'. On the other hand, there are now a number of flourishing academic centres of social medicine in Britain, a Social Medicine Research Unit of the Medical Research Council, and a Society for Social Medicine with its eponymously named journal. But it is perhaps worth noting that several of these academic departments have added the word 'preventive' to their title; and this is also true of the journal which, starting as the *British Journal of Social Medicine* in 1947, became, in 1953, the *British Journal of Preventive and Social Medicine*. One might see various implications here, but the most obvious seem to be, first, that the departments wished to emphasize an interest in *prevention*, and, second, that they did not feel – or thought that other people might not feel – that the term social medicine by itself sufficiently conveyed a concern with the prevention of disease.

PSYCHOSOCIAL MEDICINE

Soon after social medicine, and logically enough, came 'psychosocial medicine'. This was one of those terms which, though well-born and apparently healthy, seem to carry a deleterious gene. At all events, the term did not evolve further. It now survives only as the title of Dr James Halliday's brilliant book, *Psychosocial medicine* (1948), where, I suppose, it will gradually become fossilized – and a splendid fossil it will be. Halliday defined psychosocial medicine as the application of the concepts of psychosomatic medicine to the illnesses of communities and groups; and psychosomatic medicine referred, for him, to the inclusion of psychological, as well as physical, methods of investigating disease. His book is largely concerned with epidemiological studies, but its later chapters deal with the concept of 'the sick society'. By this term, of course, Halliday meant only a society so organized, or disorganized, as not to provide its members with satisfactory protection against disease. Yet the analogy is an unfortunate one. As Sir Aubrey Lewis has pointed out, the terms 'health' and 'sickness' are very difficult to define, and to extend their application from individuals to societies, other than for purely rhetorical purposes, is to confound an already confused subject.

SOCIAL PSYCHIATRY

We now approach closer to our main theme. 'Social psychiatry' is a term which, though now used in many countries, is often considered to reflect a peculiarly British contribution to our specialty. Yet the term did not originate in Britain. It appeared in the American literature as early as 1933.[1] In America, however, it remained for many years the almost exclusive property of the sociologists. Thus Dunham, addressing the American Sociological Society in 1947, says that the answer to the question 'What is social psychiatry?' is 'that it is pretty much a creation of the sociologists to designate the interest of certain of their numbers who are doing research in the field of personality disorder . . .' Dunham refers to a paper in the *American Journal of Psychiatry* for 1940, entitled 'Social psychiatry – our task or a new profession' (Hartwell, 1940), and comments: 'this is the only time to our knowledge that a psychiatrist has used the concept, "social psychiatry", and this in a context completely different from that in which the sociologists have used it' (Dunham, 1948).

In Britain, on the other hand, social psychiatry seems from the start to have been the prerogative of psychiatrists. It began to be used freely in about 1946. Thus the RMPA Section of Social Psychiatry was established at the Annual General Meeting of the Council in July that year. In 1946, too, the term was brought to the attention of a wider public by the establishment of the Institute of Social Psychiatry, under the direction of Dr Joshua Bierer. The charter of that Institute contains these words: 'In late 1946, some psychiatrists and a few laymen established the Institute in Hampstead, London. Its aspirations were to put into experimental use new methods of treatment within the social setting, and a new term, Social Psychiatry, was devised to cover this type

[1] And the term 'socio-psychiatric' occurs earlier still (Sullivan, 1931).

of work.' From this it is clear, first, that social psychiatry must have been a relatively novel phrase in Britain at that time, and, second, that in the minds of the Institute's founders, social psychiatry was a form of treatment, a form which many people might also have called group psychotherapy, or milieu therapy, or community therapy.

Now I am not, of course, going to quote all the definitions that have been given of social psychiatry. What I shall do is to make a generalization and then illustrate it. If one examines the various ways in which the term social psychiatry has been used, explicitly or implicitly, by British writers during the past twenty years, it becomes clear, I suggest, that there are two main streams of thought. Among those who attempt definitions or delimitations of social psychiatry, most give roughly the same list of activities to be included under that term; it is their emphases that differ. And the main way in which they differ is that one group emphasizes treatment and the other group emphasizes prevention. I should like to illustrate this by examining the contrasting views of two undoubted authorities.

My first authority is Dr Maxwell Jones. He was the initiator, and for twelve years the director, of the Industrial Neurosis Unit at Sutton (now called the Henderson Hospital), where his method of treatment has for many people been the example of social psychiatry *par excellence*. Recently he has become chairman of the Provisional Organizing Body of the International Association for Social Psychiatry. The Industrial Neurosis Unit at Sutton was set up in April 1947, and Dr Jones's book about its activities was published in 1952. This book was entitled *Social psychiatry*, with the subtitle, 'A study of therapeutic communities'. Dr Jones did not define or discuss the concept of social psychiatry there, but his usage is implicit in the subtitle and in the fact that the book is concerned solely with group methods of treatment. He and his colleagues conclude with the hope that they have 'contributed in some small way to the social psychiatric treatment' of their patients. Thus, in Dr Jones's concept, social psychiatry was an extension of the methods of group psychotherapy, such that staff and patients in the hospital setting formed a therapeutic community. There was nothing about prevention, or research into causes.

Dr Jones's more recent views may, I think, be taken as those expressed in a report of the World Health Organization's Expert Committee on Mental Health, the report entitled *Social psychiatry and community attitudes*, published in 1959. Here the term social psychiatry is used to refer to 'the preventive and curative measures which are directed towards the fitting of an individual for a satisfactory and useful life in terms of his own environment'. The concept has now broadened to include prevention but the emphasis is still on the measures to be taken. The nature of these measures is clearly laid down, for the report continues thus: 'In order to achieve this goal [the goal of fitting the individual for a satisfactory life], the social psychiatrist attempts to provide for the mentally ill, and for those in danger of becoming so, opportunities for making contacts with society which are favourable to the maintenance or re-establishment of social adequacy.' There is nothing here about epidemiological studies, that is, research into causes; indeed, the quotation I have just given might lead the unwary to suppose that the social causes of mental illness were already sufficiently understood. Moreover, as the measures for prevention are the same as those for treatment, there can be little distinction between the two here.

On the whole, therefore, I think that Dr Jones's concept of social psychiatry did not change much between 1952 and 1959: the emphasis is on group treatment and it has the closest relations with psychotherapy and psychodynamics. The emphasis is still on group treatment in his latest book, *Social psychiatry in the community, in hospitals and in prisons*, published in the United States in 1962. His American experience has perhaps led him to assign to psychoanalytic theory a less direct and less important role than before; but he is still not concerned with epidemiological research, and his view of preventive psychiatry still is that there is little difference between this and social therapy mainly because there are no clear boundaries between mental health and mental illness.

I now come to my second authority. Professor Sir Aubrey Lewis was the first Chairman of the Section of Social Psychiatry of the RMPA, and he was, I think, largely responsible for its receiving that name. He was also, until recently, director of the Medical Research Council's Unit for Social Psychiatry at the Maudsley Hospital. So far as I can ascertain, Professor Lewis has not made any formal definition of social psychiatry. He would probably think it unnecessary, for it seems evident from his writings on the subject that he views social psychiatry, not as a particular discipline, but simply as a term covering all the social aspects of psychiatry. Thus it covers the social causes and the social effects of mental disturbance, and the various social measures that can be taken to deal with these. For him, social psychiatry is coeval with clinical psychiatry because psychiatrists have always been interested in social factors; and he can write without any sense of anachronism about social psychiatry in the nineteenth century (Lewis, 1962). In Professor Lewis's opinion, the important change that has occurred in social psychiatry during the past two or three decades is that the study of social factors in mental disorder has become systematized and rigorous: systematized, in that particular problems are defined and investigated with the aid of techniques from sociology and epidemiology; rigorous, in that there is a willingness to put hypotheses to the chastening test of experiment and quantification, to accept the strict standards that apply in more developed fields, and not to make excuses that the subject-matter is inherently too complex for scientific method.

In his paper entitled 'Social psychiatry', published in 1956 in *Lectures on the scientific basis of medicine*, he divides his subject-matter into three parts. The first, and much the largest part, concerns *investigations* into the ways in which mental illness rates vary with cultural background, social class, marital status, migration, and so on – investigations which can be described as epidemiological. The second part deals with the *effects* of mental illness on the family and the community; the third and smallest part deals with the social aspects of *treatment* and contains a warning that the efficacy of many of our present social measures for prevention and amelioration has not yet been adequately assessed.

Two Views Compared

These, then, are the ways in which the term social psychiatry has been used by two authorities, and I suggest that they may be taken as representative in Britain of two schools of thought on the subject. If we put them side by side for a moment, we may note the following contrasts. The first school sees social psychiatry as a new discipline; the second sees it as an old one for which a new name has been found. The first school emphasizes treatment as the major activity of social psychiatry; the second emphasizes research. The first school sees the means of prevention as fundamentally the same as those of treatment; the second holds that prevention is in its infancy and that adequate measures will depend on a much greater knowledge of social causes than we have at present – hence its emphasis on research. Finally, the first school considers that social psychiatry has close links with psychotherapy and psychodynamics: the WHO Expert Committee, for example, specifically notes the indebtedness of social psychiatry to these subjects and adds that 'the goals of psychotherapy and social psychiatry can be said to overlap'; the second school sees no such links and, indeed, Professor Lewis has written that 'the claims of psycho-analysis to explain all human behaviour diverted attention from the social causes, and effects, of mental abnormality'.

Three Aspects of Social Psychiatry

I realize that I have greatly simplified, and perhaps oversimplified, a complex theme, but I now turn to consider what conclusions may be drawn from this discussion. This is not an easy matter. As Sir Francis Walshe has said, there is an urge to tidy up reality in the interests of classification. One must be on one's guard against this, and I shall not be so rash or so naïve as to press for one usage of the term social psychiatry as being better than another, or to attempt any definition of my own. I suggest, however, that the discussion permits us to draw one useful conclusion. This is that social psychiatry covers three more or less distinct types of activity.

First, there are the activities centred on, or closely associated with, the treatment of groups of patients. Activities of this kind may be called *group treatment* for short, but they comprise a range of activities from formal group psychotherapy and family psychiatry to psychiatric social clubs and therapeutic communities. Second, there are the activities concerned with increasing our knowledge of the social factors in mental disorder. This group of activities may be called *research*, and it includes epidemiological research into the causal factors of illness as well as studies designed to test the efficacy, or monitor the running, of social measures of treatment. Third, there is a group of activities, less clearly discernible because less developed, which may be called *preventive psychiatry*. It includes not only administrative and educative

measures designed to foster mental health and protect persons at
special risk, but also what has been called secondary prevention,
that is, measures to reduce the consequences of disease, such as
the provision of after-care hostels, workshops, rehabilitation
courses, and special employment facilities.

This does not exhaust the cornucopia of social psychiatry,
which has been credited to hold such other subjects as forensic
and military psychiatry. But I shall confine myself to the three
aspects that I have labelled treatment, research, and prevention;
and I now come to consider how far each of these three can expect
to find the most suitable soil for its development adjacent to the
field of psychotherapy. The test that I shall use is to see how close
are the relations of each with the methods and aims of psychotherapy. Such a test seems appropriate because, for some years
now, it has been commonly supposed that there is a close association, both in theory and in practice, between social psychiatry and
psychotherapy. Within the Royal Medico-Psychological Association, this supposition is indicated by the existence of a single
Section for Psychotherapy and Social Psychiatry. It was not always
so, for the Section was at first devoted solely to social psychiatry.
How the change occurred was mentioned in an address by Professor Lewis in 1959; I have been privileged to read the address,
which was not published, and it may be of interest if I recapitulate
the story.

In 1942, Dr P. K. McCowan, the Chairman of the Research and
Clinical Committee, asked Dr Aubrey Lewis (as he then was) to
form a subcommittee on neurosis. He agreed, but suggested that
it would be more useful if such a committee concerned itself with
the social aspects of psychiatry rather than with psychopathology
and psychotherapy 'which', to quote his words, 'were already
thoroughly discussed by other groups and associations'. This subcommittee had a vigorous life and produced various reports,
though curiously enough the more substantial of these were never
generally published. The subcommittee came to an end in May
1946, and in July of that year it was re-formed as the Section for
Social Psychiatry, with Professor Lewis as its first Chairman. He
was succeeded in 1947 by Dr J. B. S. Lewis. From this time,
psychopathological interests within the Section increased, and, in
November 1948, Dr Otto Fitzgerald, at a Council meeting, made
a plea on behalf of the Section for some means of attracting

psychotherapists to the Association. Council referred this back to the Section for a decision whether to have separate Sections for psychotherapy and for social psychiatry or to rename the Section to include both. The latter choice was made and was accepted by the Council in February 1949.

But to return from this digression to the relations of psychotherapy with the three faces of social psychiatry. It seems clear that the first of these, *treatment*, is closely allied to psychotherapy. Group therapy, community therapy, and related activities – all those aspects of social psychiatry emphasized by Dr Maxwell Jones and the WHO report – grew directly from experience of individual psychotherapy and from psychodynamic theory. The one is the child of the other, and though the child may one day grow up to leave or even to supplant its parent, I think that at present it is still best nurtured in its parental home.

With *research*, however, the relation is different. Between psychotherapy and social research there is a deep, almost a fundamental, distinction. Social research, apart from its monitoring function, aims at the uncovering of preventable causes of mental disorder and uses the methods of epidemiology. Psychotherapy is concerned with treatment, epidemiology with prevention. Psychotherapy deals with sick persons, epidemiology with populations, the sick and the healthy together. Psychotherapy is based on theories of psychopathology, but no such theories are necessary for epidemiological research. Hence, unless we are going to postulate benefit from a Jungian enantiodroma, the differences between these two subjects are so large that their close association is unlikely to be advantageous to either and may be harmful, and I therefore suggest that the epidemiological aspects of social psychiatry would develop more favourably in another soil, away from the immediate discussion and study of psychotherapy. Whether, if that happened, psychiatric epidemiology would still be thought of as part of social psychiatry, or whether it would be considered to have forsaken the shelter of that umbrella, is not, I think, a matter of any great consequence.

The relation of psychotherapy with the third aspect of social psychiatry, the *preventive* aspect, is harder to assess. It seems probable that preventive psychiatry has at present two growing-points. One focus of growth lies in group methods of treatment. It derives its inspiration and insights from psychopathological theory, and has close relations with psychotherapy; it corresponds, I think, to what has been called administrative therapy (Clark, 1965). The other focus of growth lies in the province of public health and is represented by those services – hostels, workshops, and so on – that are provided by local health authorities, or ought to be provided by them. Medical officers of mental health, and their equivalents, have not so far been numerous or active in the RMPA. I hope in time they will be, but, until then, this part of preventive psychiatry seems best represented by those research workers who try to monitor the efficiency of the public health services.

Terminological Evolution

I have dealt as best I can with the practical issues involved in the relation between psychotherapy and the different aspects of social psychiatry. I shall conclude with some comments on the practical value of the term social psychiatry. In its broad sense, meaning all the social factors in psychiatry, one might wonder if it has become so large an umbrella as to be unwieldy. In its narrow sense, there is still, after twenty years, much disagreement on the particular ground it should cover. Has it, then, any value at all?

I should like to suggest that it is – or at any rate has been – a valuable term, not so much because of any precise meaning that can be given it, as because of its function in aiding the rapid evolution of psychiatric ideas during the last twenty years. It is possible to take the view that terms like social psychiatry are terms for an occasion, developed for a special purpose, to be discarded or redeployed when this purpose has been served. In other words, they are born, run a useful but relatively short life, and then, perhaps after giving birth to better-adapted children, die. Thus one may conceive of a term introduced to cover a concept which people feel to be emerging, but which they cannot at that stage easily entrap in language, and whose direction and rate of development they cannot clearly foresee. The period of usefulness of such a term will then end when the concept has largely crystallized and is seen to have separated into several more or less well-defined blocks of interest, which should then lead independent lives under appropriate names, one of which might, of course, be the original name now captured and narrowed in meaning.

When all else is said and done, we need to remind ourselves that terminology is a matter of words and not of things. We must be on our guard against supposing that, because there is this term social psychiatry, therefore we must define it and then act in accordance with its definition. 'I am not so lost in lexicography,' said the great lexicographer, 'as to forget that words are the daughters of earth and that things are the sons of heaven.' In science, argument about the meaning of words is not necessarily profitable and may be sterilizing. Sir Cyril Hinshelwood (1965) has observed that Newton's treatment of force and mass can easily be represented as a circular argument and Einstein's spatio-temporal schemes dismissed as illogical; yet these ideas fathered nuclear energy, which no linguistic analysis can trivialize. Activities have to be subsumed under names, if only for administrative purposes; but on the principle that good wine needs no bush, the actual name probably does not matter much.

REFERENCES

ANDERSON, J. A. D. (1965). *A new look at social medicine.* London: Pitman.

CLARK, D. H. (1965). *Administrative therapy: the role of the doctor in the therapeutic community.* London: Tavistock Publications; Philadelphia: Lippincott.

DUNHAM, H. W. (1948). The field of social psychiatry. *Amer. sociol. Rev.* **13**, 183–97.

GALDSTON, I. (1954). *The meaning of social medicine.* Cambridge, Mass.: Harvard University Press.

HALLIDAY, J. L. (1948). *Psychosocial medicine.* New York: Norton; London: Heinemann, 1949.

HARTWELL, S. W. (1940). Social psychiatry – our task or a new profession? *Amer. J. Psychiat.* **96**, 1089–103.

HINSHELWOOD, C. (1965). Science and scientists. (An abridged version of the Presidential Address delivered to the British Association.) *New Scientist* **27**, 547–9.

JONES, M. (1952). *Social psychiatry: a study of therapeutic communities.* London: Tavistock/Routledge. Published in USA under the title *The therapeutic community,* New York: Basic Books, 1953.

—— (1962). *Social psychiatry in the community, in hospitals and in prisons.* Springfield, Ill.: C. C. Thomas.

c

LEWIS, A. J. (1956). Social psychiatry. In *Lectures on the scientific basis of medicine*, Vol. VI. University of London: Athlone Press; New York: Essential Books.

—— (1962). Ebb and flow in social psychiatry. *Yale J. biol. Med.* **35**, 62–83.

RYLE, J. A. (1948). *Changing disciplines*. London: Oxford University Press.

SAND, R. (1948). How medicine became social. Chadwick Public Lecture.

—— (1952). *Advance in social medicine*. Trans. R. Bradshaw. London: Staples.

SULLIVAN, H. S. (1931). Socio-psychiatric research. *Amer. J. Psychiat.* **10**, 979.

WORLD HEALTH ORGANIZATION (1959). *Social psychiatry and community attitudes*. Technical Report Series No. 177. Geneva: WHO.

2 The Issue

S. H. FOULKES

At the present time, social psychiatry is still a discipline in the making. The different ways in which various authors and factions approach it reflect faithfully the limitations and prejudices that arise in the whole field of psychiatry, in every country, between the lively, dynamic, progressive, and ever-expansive tendencies flowing from psychoanalytic sources and the limiting, conservative, static attitude, often powerfully established, tending to insist on outmoded models of 'scientific' and 'objective' verification, sometimes to the point of sterility.

Limitations and prejudices? I wish they were. In fact, deep emotional and existential attitudes, political and class factors, and much more, are involved. The same struggle permeates, on closer acquaintance, every single field of endeavour and discipline in the total culture.

In psychiatry itself this conflict becomes inevitably acute through the ever-present challenge of neurosis. The adequate response to this challenge, if it is taken seriously, can only be psychological and sociological investigation. This must take psychoanalysis and group analysis fully into account.

The antithesis between social and intrapsychic is misleading. The implication that the individual has a 'psyche', which is his innermost private self and possession, and that the social and cultural are outside forces, the individual interacting with them, is wrong, though it is a traditional notion and still reigning – often quite unconsciously.

Let us look at a relatively new discipline that has become firmly established: social psychology, especially advanced, perhaps, in the United States. Let us hear what some of its leading exponents have to say. In their classic work, *Experimental social psychology*, Murphy and Newcomb (1937) define the field as follows: 'Social psychology is the study of the way in which the individual becomes a member of, and functions in, a social group.' After stating that 'even at the level of unicellular organisms a social factor is present', they continue, 'the interaction between organisms is one of the most fundamental of biological facts'. They see the social as an aspect of the biological.

Small group research soon claimed a paramount place in the field of social psychology. In a symposium, *Group relations at the crossroads*, edited by M. Sherif and M. O. Wilson (1953), Sherif says:

'No other problem in human affairs today seems to be so crucial as that of group relations – gradually we are waking up to the realization that all these perplexing issues cannot be handled adequately without first putting them within their proper group settings. But as we study the particular group setting we begin to discover that happenings taking place there had a great deal to do with the functional relations of the group in question with other groups (intergroup relations). The conditions of social, economic, technological, cultural interdependencies between groups are there to stay. They cannot be reversed whether we like it or not.'

And later: 'The inadequacy of such one-sided approaches made an interdisciplinary approach to the study of these topics a necessity.'

Another contributor to *Group relations at the crossroads*, Herbert Blumer, puts the whole issue in a nutshell as follows: 'The premise of social psychology is that group life is the setting inside of which individual experience takes place, and that such group life exerts a decisive influence on such experience.' Given this premise, the position of social psychiatry seems clear. It is simply the pathological counterpart to social psychology, just as psychopathology is to psychology. However, as we know, it is not easy to draw a line between the normal and the abnormal. The question emerges of norm and value, in that the concept of 'normality' in a certain culture or class depends on that culture's value systems.

Some time ago I took a lady into treatment who suffered from depression, panic attacks, and phobias; she was also in the habit of drinking half a bottle of port each day. I took a different view of this last symptom when I learned that her father, with whom she was identified, was a hotelier in a Latin country.

It seems to me that social psychology and social psychiatry are two neighbouring fields – sisters – which must work hand in hand. I would presume that in laboratory and experimental work social psychology will have the upper hand, whereas, in life issues, social psychiatry will prevail.

After all, group work in small groups started with us in group psychotherapy. Our domain remains clinical research in life, experiment in action. Is that possible? I, for one, do it all day long. Dr Chance's contribution, which will be discussed later, is particularly relevant to this issue.

Another example of such experiments in life: two general practitioners, a married couple, have told me of their experience on a new housing estate near London. In one street they found a totally different incidence of illness from that in other streets, quantitatively and qualitatively, physical as well as mental disturbances. They were called many more times to this street than to others. They knew no reason for this. Could not such a phenomenon be studied systematically?

Group analysis makes full use of the social context which develops quasi-experimentally in its procedure. The patients can be observed while they interact with each other and the therapist. Experiences in this field have made it necessary to formulate new concepts both as to method and as to theory, beyond the psychological, which refer to one- and two-person situations (Foulkes, 1948, 1964; Foulkes & Anthony, 1957).

The interactional context of the group-as-a-whole is our frame of reference. What has traditionally been claimed as intrapsychic reveals itself as shareable by all the members of the group. Everything that goes on manifestly, whether in the form of symbolic representation, symptoms, or any other expression or behaviour, is considered as communication, that is to say as something to be understood and interpreted. Such understanding and interpretation occur in the first place unconsciously. The operational context of this has been termed *the group matrix*. The members of this group are, however, active participants in the process of translation on an ascending scale through which they become fully aware of all meaning. The situation just indicated, termed by me 'the group-analytic situation', is in my opinion the situation of choice for the understanding and treatment of illness as a social process.

In social psychiatry we are mainly concerned with the natural group in which the patient lives at the time of his illness and its treatment, his *network*. This is composed of the persons with whom the patient is most intimately connected, as revealed in the course of an analytical approach. As will be seen, I believe that this dynamically interacting network has a more or less fundamental significance for the production of 'illness' in an individual. Observations in the family group (Ackerman, 1958, 1961; Grotjahn, 1960) are relevant, but significant relationships are also found in the extended family and beyond. The simplest model is the triangular involvement. For instance, I have seen a number of times a husband falling in love with a foreign girl who came into the house as an *au pair* girl. The variations are great, though the marriage was in each case jeopardized and the children became neurotically involved. From whichever end of the triangle I was consulted, however, all the members of the family, and more people besides, were invariably actively involved; each one of them could have been the central patient. In these circumstances a radical total approach is often not possible, because the participants have no real wish to solve the problem. Sexual conflicts, as well as self- and other-destructive forces, are too strong, and have created conditions which make a radical approach impracticable.

We have often observed that when a significant change occurs in a patient – particularly towards greater independence – other members of the network become active. P. H. Glasser (1963) has made similar observations: The original disturbance causes disequilibrium in the family group, which is followed by a period of relief at the beginning of psychotherapy. Then comes a second period of disequilibrium. If all goes well, this is followed by a final re-equilibrium after an enforced readjustment of roles in the family members. The family is seen as a problem-solving group. Help is extended to it by auxiliary therapists, and acceptance of more limited therapeutic goals proves favourable for the results of treatment. This approach subscribes to the family's interpretation of 'the patient' as the sick member, who needs to be cured, the others not having to face their own conflicts openly.

Let us look briefly at two typical examples of networks:

Mr B, a married man of thirty, was referred for severe obsessive symptoms. He complained of being tense and keyed up, of having doubts about his actions, of having to do everything twice and to check everything. He also complained of depression and occasional wishes to die.

He had suffered from obsessional symptoms from the age of fourteen to the age of twenty, but they had eventually disappeared without treatment. Eighteen months before being referred he had been driving himself very hard at work, and gradually noted the development of his present symptoms. He felt that other people could not work with him, because he communicated tension to them, so that they had to smoke, or break off conversation with him, or complain about him.

Neat and meticulous, B had a rigid routine of living. He constantly felt himself to be in competition with others. His *mother* was reported to be very nervous, and his *mother's sister* had had the same illness as the patient, but had cured herself. The mother accompanied the patient to the hospital, stating that, naturally, she knew more about him than did his wife. She lived near them and was always in their home. She remarked that she had always seen her son in the likeness of her father; her father had suffered from a depression. The patient's father was not particularly mentioned in this connection – which was also significant.

B's relationship with his *wife* had become increasingly strained. She felt more and more shut out by her husband, and the hoped-for improvement in their relationship with the birth of a child did not materialize. They lived in close association with the wife's bachelor *uncle*. The uncle lived on the ground floor, and the wife looked after him in a kind of daughterly relationship. He was always very attached to her. He denigrated the husband's efforts at gardening, etc. The patient seemed constantly aware of this uncle's presence. Later in the drama this uncle died, but the wife's conflict became more obvious to her and she continued to mourn his death. She became aware, with surprise, of the degree of her husband's jealousy and of her own divided loyalties.

B's employers were approached. Mr G, the patient's immediate superior, turned out to be a very sympathetic and helpful person, and he indicated that he himself was of an anxious and over-conscientious disposition similar to that of the patient. He himself regularly 'took work home with him'. The managing director was less sympathetic, and afraid that G might be too much concerned with B. The patient had been very happy and competent

in his former employment until some change occurred which
involved him in travelling. The manager, who 'had his knife in
him', apparently drove him into deeper anxieties. Eventually, B
was driven into a kind of persecutory anxiety and had to leave
his employment. Since then he had never regained his confidence.

The deeper source of B's anxiety was of a castration type, and
he felt that he had lost his sense of masculinity. The marital
difficulties represented the heterosexual aspect, the work sphere
the homosexual aspect, of this disturbance. These events on the
manifest and contemporary level can be surmised to have brought
into play, and to be interacting with, the deeper levels indicated
in largely unconscious cooperation with the other participants.

Even on the basis of this merely descriptive account one can
easily discern the interaction of several classic neurotic constel-
lations. For instance, the patient's sexual disturbance was certainly
interconnected with the wife's neurosis. One might equally well
look at her as the central figure, with a typical conflict situation
between the uncle–father, the husband, and the husband's mother.

Interesting also in this case – which has been taken as a random
example – is how different essential spheres, such as work situation and family situation, come under review.

The second example is taken from a recent study at the Maudsley
Hospital, London.[1] The networks of all patients of an ordinary
ongoing therapeutic group were investigated and in every single
one of the patients a similar active network could be demonstrated. In the following instance the network under review had
been mobilized already as a result of Mr X's treatment.

X was the *brother-in-law* of the patient, Mr R. X had attended a
therapeutic group at another hospital for a number of years.
He had told R, his wife's brother, with whom he was on close
terms, a lot about this experience. It became clear that R himself,
who had never been able to approach a woman and suffered from
crippling social inhibitions generally, had been influenced by X
to seek psychotherapy for his depressing complaint.

Neither of R's parents were pleased about this. They insisted
that one should deal with life's problems oneself and not look
for help. They blamed X for everything that went wrong in the
family. X himself thought that as a result of his own treatment
the R family had come much closer together, whereas his own

marriage was breaking up. His wife, the patient's *sister*, had a fear of mental illness, related to her mother's depression, but rejected treatment. The relationship between X and R remained close and R felt that this would not change, even if X should leave the family. R was strongly fixated on his family. X said: 'R comes often to see us – seeing us quarrelling fortifies him against marrying.'

To return to R's parents: when interviewed, the *father* was very tense, at pains to emphasize his normality, but he admitted to having felt 'as though he might have an ulcer' when he recently contemplated starting a new job. His wife's depressions pre-occupied him greatly; he was active in keeping these under control, which helped him to deny his own anxiety, as often happens. She had a 'fear of being put away', and this related to his having forced her to be admitted to hospital some fifteen years ago. To his mind, her mental trouble dated from a car incident that had occurred when she was pregnant, expecting R's sister. When R left home to live on his own, this was such a shock for his mother that she had to go back to hospital for further treatment: 'She needs her son.'

The *mother* herself said that she had been quite unaware, until R left home, that anything troubled him. Her children had 'always seemed quite normal'. Since starting treatment R had talked much more openly to them and had told her things of which she was unaware. A major theme in her life was an attempt to make up for the lack of love she felt had been her lot through the experiences of her children.

It will have become clear that R had changed in the course of his treatment in the direction of greater independence and social freedom, precipitating the mother's reaction. R himself expressed at that time in his treatment a fear that his mother would think that he had no right to attend.

This second example is an abbreviated account of a network which was dynamically investigated. In all these individuals who were not otherwise selected, who had in common only that they had been referred for psychotherapy at the Maudsley Hospital and had been found suitable for group psychotherapy, equally active networks could be clearly demonstrated. The details of these networks provided a fascinating variety, and it is hoped to publish this study more fully. In the group-analytic view, the processes operate and interact in the total psychodynamic field of the network group, its matrix, passing, as it were, right through the individuals of this group in a manner that might be compared to x-rays. Hence I prefer to speak not merely of interactional processes between individuals, but of *transpersonal* processes.

Illness and related disturbances are due to psychopathological processes which thus involve a number of interrelated persons. The individual can be seen as a participant in a drama. In the psychoneuroses this *multipersonal network of interaction* is of central significance. Change in any one member of such a network is linked to changes in other members of that network. I have been impressed increasingly over the years by observations which seem to show that even the nature of an individual's symptoms, or other manifestations of tension, rest on this interdependence (Foulkes, 1948, 1964; Foulkes & Anthony, 1957). This group of interrelated persons, e.g. the family group, should always be considered as the framework for diagnosis and prognosis, even where a simultaneous approach to the whole group is not practicable.

Illness emerges as a social, interpersonal process. Its psycho-social analysis is of particular value in bringing to light the concealed meaning and significance of the many guises in whice illness appears. It furnishes a key, in particular, to the approach to *unconscious processes* in three areas:

> the personal, repressed meaning, based on the original family group, in psychoanalysis;
> the unconscious, interpersonal interaction, the 'social unconscious', in group analysis;
> the society's ills, and thus the unconscious origins of much human behaviour.

The foregoing observations and examples should indicate clearly enough why it is my opinion that psychotherapy and, in particular, group psychotherapy – especially that developed on a psychoanalytic foundation and the techniques deriving from it – are of absolutely central importance for practice and research in social psychiatry.

The opposite view is well represented by Dr Hare, who has given us an interesting account, also from a historical perspective. If one accepts his definitions, he has made a good case for a separate and safe Section for research. Research is seen as incompatible with treatment: ' . . . no [psychopathological] theories are necessary for epidemiological research.' And, 'Between psychotherapy and social research there is a deep, almost a fundamental, distinction.' It is almost as if Dr Hare feels that social psychiatry would be contaminated by contact with psychotherapy. He is in this respect in strong contrast to many modern sociologists, such as Talcott Parsons and Elias.

What we are left with is a social psychiatry that consists of sociological research into psychiatric issues. Psychotherapy, group psychotherapy, community therapy, and administrative therapy are all laudable activities, but they must not be mixed up with social psychiatry. The philosophy behind this concept of social psychiatry is that of an impartial science, incompatible with participation in or motivation for change. There is no question of the value of such research for all of us, so far as it can be realized. These studies form, so to speak, our anatomy, but anatomy is not enough.

For such an approach all concepts must be static. There are, for instance, 'diseases' with their natural history, which, as it were, fall upon a person who suffers from them. By contrast, in our view, psychiatry is concerned with people suffering from maladaptations, from conflicts internal and external, which they cannot solve as well as they might. There is also, of course, a static concept of science itself as an objective approach based on statistical, measurable, and mathematical statements. It has long been shown and understood in the exact sciences, for example physics, that these concepts are out of date. It has been universally recognized that we cannot examine anything or experiment with anything without changing the situation and without introducing the observer himself. In this sense Freud's psychoanalysis is a much better model of modern science than is the classical outdated concept of physics (see Hutten, 1962).

The difference between our two approaches has been characterized as that between *objective* psychiatry and *personal* psychiatry. The latter is a dynamic pursuit, entailing involvement and change in one's own person, and threatening values and attitudes. There is resistance against such change. The techniques of segregation, isolation, detachment, and non-involvement are clearly preferred.

The main difference between the approach advocated here and that of Dr Hare is, however, that the former considers the social not as external, but as internally represented. The social and cultural matrix enters deeply into the very structure of the personality. I should like to quote a little from the Kinsey report (Kinsey *et al.*, 1948), a report that certainly lives up to the standards of a 'scientific' and statistical investigation. Let us hear what Kinsey has to say:

> 'The quality of a case history study begins with the quality of the interviewing by which the data have been obtained. . . . Learning how to meet people of all ranks and levels, establishing rapport, sympathetically comprehending the significances of things as others view them, learning to accept their attitudes and activities without moral, social, or esthetic evaluation, being interested in people as they are, and not as someone else would have them, learning to see the reasonable bases of what at first glance may appear to be most unreasonable behavior, developing a capacity to like all kinds of people and thus to win their esteem and cooperation – these are the elements to be mastered by one who would gather human statistics' (p. 35).

> 'These social levels are, admittedly, intangible divisions of the population which are difficult to define; but they are recognized by everyone as real and significant factors in the life of a community' (p. 329).

Throughout his book Kinsey shows that sexual behaviour at different social levels is strikingly different even in the same city or town, and sometimes in immediately adjacent sections of the community:

> 'The data show that divergencies in the sexual patterns of such social groups may be as great as those which anthropologists have found between the sexual patterns of different racial groups in remote parts of the world' (p. 329).

The Kinsey report is one of the many documents from various fields in recent times which have shown, beyond doubt, that all values, e.g. what is normal and what is abnormal, are determined by the culture in which the events take place. This is true not only for different cultures but even for different social classes within the same town or even the same neighbourhood (see Elias & Scotson, 1965). Such findings have far-reaching consequences. In the field of sexual behaviour in particular, what is normal and what is abnormal are also strongly connected with moral evaluation, and to sin against the standards of the community or the class (far more than against the law itself) has disastrous consequences for the individual. The standards of the upper classes are so different from those of the lower classes that they are almost diametrically opposed. It is common knowledge in certain courts in the United States that a judge who comes from the upper strata will condemn certain delinquents far more severely than will a judge who comes from the lower-middle class, and vice versa. This is so well known that social workers and solicitors see to it that their cases come up at a favourable date.

The problems arising, as presented in this volume, are certainly psychiatric ones. The psychiatrist must be familiar with them, since he is, or should be, the person best equipped to be called upon as consultant in respect of the resultant diseases. This is dangerous ground for him, however. The borderline between healthy and sick disappears. The art of interviewing and the attitudes required as fundamental for the social scientist are exactly the same as those cultivated by the psychotherapist. Psychotherapy in turn becomes a social science. Interest in the group with me, for example, came not as an outgrowth from individual psychoanalysis, merely as another technique. My interest in the operational and conceptual area of the group was the consequence of the insight that neurosis itself must be seen as a multipersonal manifestation.

Group analysis is not the child of psychoanalysis; this is only historically true. It is, in fact, a more comprehensive approach which does or should comprise individual psychoanalysis. Psychoneurosis and allied disturbances grow from the family, they are symptoms of disturbed family life; later, they grow from the extended family, or the 'network of interaction', in my terminology. The family itself, however, is deeply imbued with and totally conditioned by the values of its surrounding culture and the reflection of this culture in the particular class to which it belongs.

Group treatment, group-analytic treatment, and group-analytic study have long since proved valuable tools of investigation and teaching, apart from their value for therapy. This is exactly because one can see changes and their consequences, as in an experiment under one's own eyes. We are interested in change and in the study of change. This is just as well, because we live in a world of rapid change, which is the point of departure of this volume. It is the reason why, over a whole year, various experts were asked to talk to psychiatrists.

Reports of current troubles in various spheres will be the future psychiatrist's case conference. From this material he will learn to listen, analyse, and diagnose. On the basis of family and other network-group investigations he will better understand the roots of his individual patients' ailments, whether he treats these individuals alone or within the social context of a small group.

The most relevant scientific contributions may come from experimental, though not necessarily artificial, situations. They will concern the study of *change in operation*, the study of change in a living situation.

NOTE

1. This study was supported by a grant from the Research Committee of the Institute of Psychiatry, University of London.

REFERENCES

ACKERMAN, N. W. (1958). *The psychodynamics of family life: diagnosis and treatment of family relationships*. New York: Basic Books.

—— (1961). Symptom, defense, and growth in group process. *Int. J. Gp. Psychother.* **2**.

BLUMER, H. (1953). In Sherif & Wilson (see below).

ELIAS, N. & SCOTSON, J. L. (1965). *The established and the outsiders*. London: Frank Cass.

FOULKES, S. H. (1948). *Introduction to group-analytic psychotherapy*. London: Heinemann.

—— (1964). *Therapeutic group analysis*. London: Allen & Unwin; New York: International Universities Press, 1965.

—— & ANTHONY, E. J. (1957). *Group psychotherapy*. Harmondsworth: Penguin Books. Revised edn, 1965.

GLASSER, P. H. (1963). Changes in family equilibrium during psychotherapy. *Family Process* **2**.

GROTJAHN, M. (1960). *Psychoanalysis and the family neurosis.* New York: Norton.

HUTTEN, E. H. (1962). *The origins of science.* London: Allen & Unwin.

KINSEY, A. C. *et al.* (1948). *Sexual behavior in the human male.* Philadelphia, Pa.: W. B. Saunders.

MURPHY, G. & NEWCOMB, T. M. (1937). *Experimental social psychology.* New York: Harper.

SHERIF, M. & WILSON, M. O. (eds.) (1953). *Group relations at the crossroads.* New York: Harper.

Part II: Problems Encountered in Communities and Institutions

3 Psychosis and Social Change among the Tallensi of Northern Ghana

MEYER FORTES and DORIS Y. MAYER

I CULTURAL AND SOCIAL CONTEXT

The investigation we report in this paper relates to the Tallens of Northern Ghana. It falls into three sections. In the first two, contributed by M.F., the cultural and social context of the inquiry is sketched and the observations which directly stimulated our inquiry are reported. In the third, the psychiatric observations made by D.Y.M. in 1963 are described and discussed. Thirty years ago I carried out an intensive anthropological study of this tribal society over a period of two and a half years. In 1963, a generation later, my wife, Dr Doris Mayer, and I spent about three months among the Tallensi.[1] At the time of my first visit they were hardly affected by Western ideas and ways of life. British rule had brought peace and more security than they had previously enjoyed. A fair sprinkling of the younger men were already making a practice of going (what was for them) 'abroad', that is, to the Southern cocoa and mining areas three to four hundred miles away, to work for wages; but most of them went for short spells and quickly fell back into the traditional economic and social environment on their return.[2] There were no Christian missions, or

[1] The fieldwork on which this paper is based was carried out in Northern Ghana during the period September to December 1963. It was made possible by a personal grant originally given to one of us (M.F.) by the Behavioral Sciences Division of the Ford Foundation. We acknowledge this assistance with gratitude. We are greatly indebted, also, to the government of Ghana, in the persons, particularly, of the Regional Commissioner for the Upper Region and his Secretary and staff, for the encouraging interest they took in our research but even more for the material facilities placed at our disposal. Without these we should have had to give up before we got started.

[2] From the inquiries I made in 1934–37, it appeared that about one in three of the adult males had at some time or another visited or worked in what is

33

dispensaries, or administrative offices, and no schools, in the tribal area, the nearest being some ten miles away in the neighbouring Gorensi area. There was only a handful – four or five – of literate Tallensi youths in the area. There were no bicycles or ploughs and it was only in the houses of the half-dozen or so richer chiefs and headmen that one saw such articles of foreign manufacture as buckets and kerosene lamps, which had usually been brought back from the South by returned labour migrants.

I should add that I lived in close contact with the people, spoke their language quite fluently, and knew intimately many families and individuals, especially in the central community of Tongo which was my headquarters.

The Traditional Social Structure

I have described the social structure and mode of life of the Tallensi as I knew them a generation ago in a number of publications,[1] but some account of the salient features, comparing conditions at that time with the present social and cultural circumstances of the people, is necessary to give perspective to our discussion. The most striking immediate impression made on me after an absence of thirty years was of the basic stability, up to the present time, of their social organization and way of life, in the face of many changes. The Tallensi are typical of a congeries of tribes who speak closely related dialects of the same language family and have very close affinities in their economic, political, domestic, and religious institutions and customs. They live in the savannah zone of Northern Ghana and adjacent territories. They numbered between thirty and forty thousand in the 'thirties and now number about fifty thousand.[2] They do not live in compact villages but in family homesteads standing separately at short distances from one another and spreading endlessly over the flat countryside. At the border with their neighbours, the Gorensi, homesteads of the two groups intermingle. They are indeed so

now Southern Ghana. However, only about 7 per cent of the total adult male population were estimated to be more or less permanently away from their home communities. The 'culture-contact' situation of that period is briefly described in Fortes (1936).

[1] See, in particular, Fortes (1945, 1949, 1959).

[2] This is a rough estimate based on the census of 1960.

much alike in culture that outsiders cannot distinguish between them.

This country is very densely settled. Dry to the point of aridity in the six months of the dry season (October to April), it is lush with the staple crops of millet and sorghum during the rainy season from April to September in a normal year. The basis of social organization throughout the area is the patrilineal clan and lineage with a founding ancestor placed some fourteen generations back; and there can be little doubt that the people have been sedentary here for at least the two to three hundred years represented in their genealogies.

Grain-farming was formerly and still is the principal source of livelihood for the tribe. Each family group farms for itself and tends its own livestock, thus being almost wholly self-supporting. But it was and remains a marginal economy. Nowadays money, mostly earned in Southern Ghana, contributes appreciably to the income of many families. For the majority, nevertheless, the standard of living still leaves no surplus over needs. Farming is subject to hazards of climate which, until recently, often resulted in periods of near-starvation. Men do the heavy work, women assist with the lighter tasks such as harvesting. Women also take care of the home, which is arduous enough. Preparing food, bringing in the firewood and water, keeping the home clean, and attending to the needs of the young children add up to a heavy schedule. In the 'thirties, boys and girls from the age of about seven years helped in these economic tasks. Nowadays many[1] attend the local schools or are away at secondary boarding schools. Older people complain of the disruption that has been caused in the traditional farming system by, for example, the lack of herd-boys for their cattle, though the increasing use of ox-drawn ploughs in place of hand-hoeing has reduced the need for labour on the land. Population increase, though not as heavy as in many other parts of Africa, and mitigated as it is by the opportunities for labour migration to the South, is also a factor in this penurious economy. And to these external pressures must be added the hazards of tropical and other diseases.

---

[1] A rough survey made in 1963 suggested that well over half the boys aged six to sixteen approximately were attending school and around one-third of the girls. In a sample of fifty-two families, only one with children of school age had none at school.

The Family System

Yet acutely aware as they are of these sources of insecurity, the Tallensi did not formerly and do not now give the impression of living with a constant feeling of threat hanging over their heads. This is due, to no small extent, to their family system. In this domain, their social life has remained unchanged since my first visit. A striking sign of the stability of their family system is the fact that the siting and distribution of homesteads in my base community of Tongo were in 1963 exactly the same as they had been in 1937. Some had been enlarged to accommodate family segments which had proliferated during this period, and some were smaller as a result of decline in family size. A few new homesteads had been built but these were all on old family sites.

The Tallensi have one of the most consistent patrilineal and patriarchal family systems as yet observed in Africa. At the peak of the cycle of family development (cf. Fortes, 1958) the homestead is normally occupied by a family group consisting of an old man, his adult sons and possibly his sons' sons, together with the wives of these men and all their unmarried children. This is the ideal every man aims at. Three-generation patrilineal, polygynous families are common. By the rule of lineage exogamy, daughters marry out. Men are born, grow up, and live their lives in the same place and often homestead. Even if they spend many years working in Southern Ghana they can and normally do return freely to their natal home when they wish to do so. Women live in their parental home as daughters and move to their husbands' homes as wives; and though the physical distance of the move may be less than a mile, the social distance is felt to be significant. Furthermore, the men of a lineage united by ties of common patrilineal descent which go back many generations tend to live near one another. Since, by the rules of classificatory kinship, they are all 'brothers', 'fathers', and 'sons' to one another, the feeling of family solidarity embraces a whole cluster of kinship-linked parental families, each of which, however, has its separate house or part of a house. Thus the core of every community is a group of patrilineally linked men, and it is they who hold the reins of authority and power in regard to land and livestock, and the control of women and children, and especially in regard to the all-important religious cult of ancestor worship.

At the same time women have a remarkable degree of autonomy. Throughout life they keep in close touch with their own parental kinsfolk. Indeed, as among other African patrilineal peoples, the mother's brother plays an important part in a person's life as the indulgent, protective non-authoritarian counterpoise to the father and paternal kin. A wife with children is entitled to have her own apartment which is the private domain of herself and her children. The mother's room, both in reality and in the imagery and conceptualization of family structure, is the heart of the family. Sexual relations between husband and wife are prohibited from the time of a baby's birth until he can run about and feed himself. Thus children are normally spaced at three-yearly intervals, approximately, and immediately successive matri-siblings are believed and expected to have strong feelings of rivalry, which they often display in early childhood.

From a child's point of view, then, his life-space falls into a series of zones, corresponding to successive stages of development. The innermost zone is centred on his mother and her room; next comes the zone of the father-centred homestead associated with the ideas of half-siblingship and of paternal authority; and then, operative increasingly after the age of about five, the cluster of related families. A contrapuntal pattern of social organization, in which patrilateral and matrilateral relationships are balanced against each other, is fundamental in all spheres of Tallensi social structure and personal attitudes. It has not changed perceptibly during the past thirty years. Attachment to the family and respect for the father remain so strong that educated young men working as clerks, teachers, etc. continue to live in their parental home and to contribute to the family income just as their fathers did before them.

But I must not leave a wrong impression. 'Patriarchy' and 'patriliny' are words that carry overtones of an authoritarian family pattern. Among the Tallensi, the remarkable stability of their family system in the face of quite significant social changes is, I think, to no small degree due to the very benevolent character of their form of patriarchy. This comes out most obviously in the upbringing of infants and young children. Men and women take equal delight, and show equal affection and indulgence, in looking after their young children. Corporal punishment is very rare. Obedience to parents is built into the domestic routine and the value system rather than enforced by coercion. Individuals, even quite young children, have a large measure of independence within the framework of duty to the family.[1]

A notable aspect of Tallensi culture is the way in which the family system is mirrored and sanctioned in the ancestral cult. The shrines dedicated to the departed ancestors are placed all over the homestead; and when not receiving sacrifice or worship are quite informally used as tables or seats. This shows vividly how the ancestors continue to form part of the family almost as if they were still among the living. They have in fact been reincorporated in the family in their spiritual identity. Essentially, all ancestors worshipped are translated parents. Both paternal and maternal ancestors are thus worshipped. All ancestor figures are invested with mystically punitive as well as (but rather more than) beneficent qualities; but, significantly enough, maternal ancestors and ancestresses, who are extensions of the loving and self-sacrificing mother to whom unqualified affection and trust are due, are believed to be more vindictive than are paternal ones, who represent the respected and legally supreme father. From the point of view of their descendants, the ancestors are perpetually demanding recognition, service, and propitiation by means of libations and blood sacrifices, claiming the credit for a person's good fortune and, more usually, asserting their rights by inflicting misfortune, sickness, and above all death.[2] Being unpredictable, their intervention gets known only after the event, when a diviner is consulted to discover the ancestral agent of an illness or a death. As we shall see, though, madness is an exception to this pattern.

I will not venture on a psychological interpretation of Tallensi ancestor worship. I will only remark that in one respect the ancestors can be seen as the projection, in symbol and concept, of the coercive authority and superior power that lie behind the

---

[1] These traditional patterns are described in Fortes (1949). Their persistence, to judge by our observations in 1963, is additional testimony to the strength of Tallensi family structure. School attendance has not perceptibly affected the relations of parents with their infant children. Such traditional customs as the post-partum bathing of mother and babe are firmly adhered to, as are the traditional patterns of family etiquette. Nor, indeed, have there been noticeable changes in the relations between parents and older children. As one informant remarked, 'It is because our children still respect us in the same way as we did our parents that we don't object to their going to school.'
[2] I discuss this aspect of Tallensi ancestor worship at length in Fortes (1959).

affection and devotion of parents (especially fathers) for their children. In another, ancestor worship may be seen as a mechanism for dealing with the ambivalence in the relations of parents and children that Tallensi custom openly recognizes. For example, a man and his first-born son and prospective heir are deemed to be rivals and are therefore obliged to avoid certain forms of intimate contact; and a similar rule applies in an attenuated form to a woman and her oldest daughter. Furthermore, a man does not achieve the status of full jural independence until his father dies, no matter what his age may be.

I must add that it would be quite wrong to imagine the Tallensi as living in constant dread of their ancestors. In some ways ancestors are much like small children or very old people, noticed only when they make a nuisance of themselves by their demands or by getting ill. Then they must be placated and one can relax until the next outburst.

Tallensi thought is so dominated by the belief in the supremacy of the departed ancestors that there is little room for other supernatural forces in their cosmology. Supernatural power matching that of the ancestors is attributed to the Earth. But witchcraft and sorcery, so prominent in other indigenous African religions, for example among the Akan peoples of Southern Ghana[1] and among the Yoruba of Nigeria,[2] are marginal in the Tallensi system of belief. The essence of witchcraft and sorcery is that they are maleficent superhuman powers believed to be lodged in or employed by one's living fellow men, most often, in Africa, kinsfolk or neighbours. The idea of this power exists in Tallensi thought, but it has a role rather like that of the idea of ghosts or of premonitory dreams among ourselves. In the test case of serious illness or death, the final cause is invariably the ancestors, or their personified ally the Earth, never a witch or sorcery. Indeed, in the case of death, if neither ancestors nor the Earth claim to have caused it, the deceased is believed never to have been really human.

The demands and the claims of ancestors are made known through a diviner. Divination among the Tallensi, in keeping with their generally realistic outlook, is a matter-of-fact business, conducted with the aid of a collection of mnemonic objects. Mediumistic divination by shamans or by priests in a state of possession,

---

[1] As described, for instance, in Field (1960).
[2] Cf. Prince (1964).

as practised, for example, among the Ashanti of Southern Ghana,[1] is unheard of and completely alien to the Tallensi. Tallensi who have seen such forms of divination and doctoring in Southern Ghana speak of them with scorn. The notion of possession by the spirit of a departed ancestor, a deity, or any other supernatural agency is, indeed, inconceivable to them.

The fact is that Tallensi culture is fundamentally mundane. They do not divide the universe into a natural and a supernatural sphere. The ancestors are integrally part of their social organization. Magical power is lodged in real and tangible objects. Tallensi have occasion enough for fear, anxiety, and grief, and they take it for granted that people are moved by greed, lust, envy, and malice. But they regard these as moral failings not as sins. And it is fully in accord with this mundane attitude to the world and to human relationships that they strike an observer as singularly free of overt reactions of guilt and remorse. The reason is, I believe, not far to seek. The psychological roots of these attitudes probably go back to the benign child-rearing practices of the people. Their institutional support lies in the relationship of the living with their dead ancestors. The ancestors are the keepers of conscience; and since they are so palpable and approachable by customary ritual, the offences against them to which grave misfortunes are generally attributed can be put right by propitiatory sacrifices or other religious observances.

I am referring, of course, to situations of crisis or stress beyond the reach of the normal resources of knowledge and skill provided by Tallensi traditional culture – for example, the failure of a man's crops, the serious sickness of wife or child, a death in the family, and so forth. In the affairs of practical life, the Tallensi impressed me, when I was first among them, by their high standards of honesty and responsibility. Even nowadays, according to information given to us by the local magistrate, cases of theft are extremely rare in the Tallensi area. So also are cases of assault. Those that arise are almost invariably due to brawls in the market place among men who have been drinking. Again, one need only talk to some of the two hundred or so mothers who come crowding around the weekly child-care clinic nowadays conducted by the nearby Presbyterian mission to realize what a strong sense of responsibility Tallensi have. Some of these mothers walk a dozen

[1] Cf. Field (1960, *passim*).

miles to bring an ailing child in to be seen by the nurse. I do not want to imply that Tallensi are less prone than the majority of mankind to try to get round the law when it suits their convenience. But, by and large, they are conscientious in meeting their obligations in the affairs of everyday life.

Questions of overt guilt and remorse do not arise in these situations. In my view, the main reason why they are, so to speak, side-tracked in situations of crisis is that the reactions of the dead ancestors to human conduct are quite unpredictable. One fails in one's religious duties to them unwittingly rather than knowingly. Thus when a disaster happens one learns only after the event how one has been remiss, and one can make reparation in the prescribed ritual way without feeling guilty or remorseful.[1] I might add, in passing, that these religious and moral ideas and values have lost none of their hold on the people. A Catholic mission is now at work in the tribal area, and other missions have also been busy, especially among Tallensi schoolchildren and older literates. But there is as yet only a handful of adult converts and they are all still too junior in age and status to have any influence in the conduct of family and community affairs.

Notions of Illness

Tallensi notions of the nature and causes of illness and their methods of treatment need some consideration here. An illness is named by reference to the part of the body most affected, but there is a vague notion that all forms of illness are manifestations of disorder either in the head or in the belly or in both – with good reason perhaps, in view of the prevalence of malaria and dysentery. Illness is ingrained in the human constitution. Normally dormant, it rises up when evoked. Exposure to cold or the sun may stir up a passing fever, and eating unripe crops may cause diarrhoea. Such minor maladies are treated with home remedies. What precipitates serious illnesses such as dysentery or pneumonia is a mystery; but their ultimate cause is believed to be non-material. The ancestors are first in line. They may inflict illness and its consequence, death, in punishment for disregard of kinship duties, for breach of taboo, above all for neglect, witting or not, of their claims. But they may act also by withdrawing their protection and leaving the way open to other occult agents of misfortune. The

[1] This subject is dealt with at length in Fortes (1959).

most important and dangerous of these are magically 'evil' animals, 'evil' trees, and 'evil' stones – not, be it noted, evil people. If a man kills a big game animal he must be immediately cleansed by treatment with the proper medicine lest the victim prove to be an evil animal whose spirit will try to harm him.

Evil trees and stones, being more ubiquitous and accessible, are more sinister. As we shall see, they are particularly connected with madness. Interestingly enough, they are also dangerous to young infants and post-partum women. Babies wear protective charms to fend off these enemies whose attacks would cause them to develop an incurable wasting disease.

It is to be noted that these evil trees and stones are not only non-human but a-human. There are mystically good trees and good stones. These are believed to be the material vehicles of ancestor spirits or the powers of the Earth. As such they are within the scheme of moral relationships generated in the family and embracing the ancestors. The evil trees and stones are not, and are therefore not amenable to propitiation by the normal rituals of worship and sacrifice. It is true that, since they are personified, attempts may be made to placate them by offerings and invocations. But the attitude here is that such action may induce them to desist. It is not meant to gain their goodwill. Just how these trees and stones exercise their malign powers is not clearly explained by the Tallensi. They act out of sheer malice, without the justifiable motives that are attributed to ancestors whose authority has been flouted or whose service has been neglected. It is said that they sometimes change into humans, taking on the shape of a kinsman or a stranger. They then approach their victim and solicit food or drink, in a kind of parody of the way in which ancestors demand sacrifices. If they are denied, they attack their victim and derange his mind. This is thought of as an external assault, not, be it noted, as a kind of possession. It implies, of course, that the protection of the ancestors has been withdrawn from the victim, though they are not the direct agents of his injury. It implies, also, that though he has been trapped by deceit, he is in some degree personally at fault for flouting the most elementary norms of amity in social relationships.

Treatment follows the standard pattern of Tallensi magico-herbal medicine. It is carried out in the patient's home. A man who owns the appropriate medicine is summoned. He brings his roots and herbs, boils some in water and burns some to powder, performs the necessary sacrifices, and prescribes the standard treatment: the patient is bathed with the infusion, drinks some of it and is given the powder in his food, daily, for a fixed (usually three for a man and four for a woman) number of days. In the case of madness, this part of the treatment may be preceded by searching out with the aid of a diviner the actual tree or stone believed to have caused the madness, and attempting to placate it by offering it the food and drink it was supposed to have been denied by the victim.

The diviner, incidentally, is a key person in tracing the mystical agent of illness and death. No one can deduce for himself which of the many ancestors to whom he owes religious services or what other mystical agent, be it the Earth or an evil tree or stone, is responsible for his or his dependant's illness or death. This can be established only by divination.

To provide treatment for sick dependants is one of the most binding duties of a family head, evasion of which brings down the wrath of the ancestors. Tallensi, like people all over the world, never lose hope and often try doctor after doctor. Family solidarity, moreover, enlists the hopes and support of a wide range of kin in the treatment of the sick. That is why the families of my wife's patients took such lively interest in her endeavours to help them. But in a case of chronic madness, Tallensi soon realize and sadly accept that a cure is probably impossible, and reconcile themselves, as best may be, to putting up with the unfortunate sufferer.

These traditional beliefs concerning illness and the methods of treatment associated with them still prevail among the majority of the people. But one big change, since I first lived among the Tallensi, is in their attitudes to European medicine. They are now familiar with our pills and injections and are eager to have the benefit of them. Lepers are very regular in attendance at the weekly leper clinic to receive their medicine. The sick are often taken to the hospital at Bolgatanga, ten miles away, if they are mobile or transport happens to be available. The clerks and teachers and other literates, as well as the more sophisticated non-literate men and women who have had experience of medical treatment in the South, seem now to have no respect left for the traditional forms of treatment of common diseases, and their example is, in this matter, influential. But most of them still accept the theory of the ultimate mystical causation of illness and death – be it ancestors for the non-Christians or God for the Christians – and take the attitude of submission to the inevitable in the face of such misfortune.

Recent Social Change

I have stressed the stability of the family structure of the Tallensi and the continuity of their basic religious and magical ideas over the past thirty years. But there have been many significant changes in their social order, too. I have already mentioned that a large proportion of the children now go to school, that a Catholic mission is active in the Tallensi area, that an elite of young literates is emerging. It is a sign of the changed times that one now never sees young girls and unmarried maidens going about in public in the proud nudity which was the custom a generation ago, though many older women still go about their daily work clothed only in the perineal waistband of traditional matronhood. Very few men, and these only the elderly, now go about in the traditional garb of a loincloth and a sheep or goat skin. Another sign of the changed times and of the generally increased level of prosperity in this area is the prevalence of the bicycle. On a rough estimate, somewhat over a half of all the families in the Tongo area now have at least one bicycle each. In 1937, mine was the only one in this area. This invaluable vehicle has greatly increased the mobility of the people and the range of their contacts. Bicycles and passenger lorries make it easy to frequent the rapidly growing and cosmopolitan urban centre and market town of Bolgatanga ten miles away, with its stores selling imported wares, its lorry park, and its poky bars, as well as its schools, hospital, and modern suburban development.

Economically, the Tallensi still largely rely on subsistence farming. A bad harvest can create a food shortage, though facilities for buying imported maize and other foodstuffs mitigate the worst effects. But a money economy is now firmly fixed on top of the subsistence pattern. This means that their economy now benefits substantially from money earned abroad and remitted home, to a degree that was not experienced thirty years ago. A large proportion of the younger men, as I have mentioned, probably even the majority of them,[1] now work periodically in Southern Ghana, and many spend many years there. At the same time, the excellent roads and mail services enable them to keep in regular touch with the home community. Visits to and from Southern Ghana are frequent; letters pass back and forth; and imported goods of all kinds, as well as money, thus percolate to the home community.

New occupations, new tastes, and new goals are emerging within the Tallensi area, though as yet on a small scale, in consequence of these external economic and social contacts. Apart from teachers and clerks, petty traders, one or two quite big dealers in livestock, and a few artisans represent these new occupations. A new taste is catered for in the distillation and sale, now legally permitted, of crude gin. In 1963 it seemed to have become quite a common beverage on occasions both of private hospitality and of public celebration. This innovation was deplored by most of the older people who remain faithful to the traditional, and comparatively innocuous, millet and guinea-corn beer. Some of the cases of madness to be described later were blamed directly on excessive gin-drinking. New goals are linked with the possibilities opened up by education, by new occupational outlets, by work abroad, by wage- and salary-earning at home, and so forth. Though still limited in range, all these developments point to the emergence of new patterns of living in the near future.

In other words, the social, economic, and cultural horizons have expanded enormously in thirty years. People are more aware of the outside world. The clerks, teachers, and school and college boys coming home for their vacations, kept up to date by means of their radios and the newspapers, spread news about other parts of the country and distant lands. Political officials making propaganda speeches constantly emphasize national rather than local ideals. National political movements and changes have struck at the heart of the old order of tribal political structure even in the much reduced form it had thirty years ago. Chiefs and clan heads have been deprived of their former power and authority to settle disputes and organize communal activities. What vestiges of

---

[1] The figures from the 1960 census are difficult to interpret. My own rough estimate, based on the inquiries I made in November 1963, is that well over half of the men aged twenty to fifty who would normally be living at home were then working in Southern Ghana or elsewhere outside the tribal area.

authority they retain are exercised *sub rosa* and it is widely alleged
that corruption is common among them. Thus the traditional
sense of clan solidarity and of the interdependence of neighbouring clans is very much diminished.

These structural changes have brought in their train a
loosening-up of the traditional value system. In the setting of the
changing cultural environment, the effect is to confront people
with problems of choice not hitherto encountered. Take the case
of D.B. He is an intelligent, well-paid clerk living at home in his
father's house, but in his own quarters. For months he was in a
state of mounting psychological turmoil. On the one hand he felt
bound, by his genuine loyalty and affection for his father and his
sense of family solidarity, to contribute substantially to the family
exchequer. On the other, he wanted to use his earnings to improve
his own living quarters and to buy clothes and other items of
property that go with the status of an educated man, and he
therefore resented the demands made by his father. In practice,
this came down to choosing how to allocate his monthly salary
without offence to his father. It was a dilemma of a kind that
could not have arisen thirty years ago.

To sum up, the more or less self-contained traditional society
that I knew so well in the middle 'thirties is now wide open. The
impression is inescapable, when I cast my mind back for comparison, that the Tallensi are at a critical point of transition in their
social history. Their traditional social structure and way of life
are on the brink of far-reaching transformation.

In regard, more particularly, to their family system, formerly it
was integrated with the wider society by bonds of kinship,
marriage, neighbourhood, and religious association – the same
bonds, in fact, that bind its members together internally. What
seems to be emerging now is a distinct cleavage and incompatibility between, on the one hand, the still relatively stable, traditionally constituted, patrilineal family in its internal organization and
value system, and, on the other, the external social, economic, and
ideological sphere in which individual members of a family can
play a role divorced from traditional norms – with side-effects on
their family relations of the kind illustrated in the case of D.B.
This seems to be a very recent development, going back some ten
years at the most. It is significant that in the majority of my wife's
cases psychotic breakdown was associated with experiences under-

gone in this extra-familial sphere of social life, whether in the urbanized and alien South or even at home. This is where the stresses in modern conditions that precipitate mental illness among a tribal people like the Tallensi emanate from.

II MENTAL ILLNESS AMONG THE TALLENSI, 1934–1937

Some General Considerations

I want to go back now to the observations that led up to the present investigation. At the time when I first went out to work among the Tallensi, there was already a ferment of discussion, originally inspired by Freud's *Totem and taboo*, concerning the apparent parallels between customary beliefs and practices found in primitive societies and psychopathological conditions met with in our own society. In particular, my teacher and friend the late Professor C. G. Seligman, a pioneer of psychological anthropology in Great Britain, drew attention to the cross-cultural problems of psychosis (Seligman, 1929, 1932). To begin with, there was and is the question of what similarities or differences exist, on the one hand, in the manifestations of mental illness and, on the other, in their incidence, in different types of social system and cultural tradition. And, second, there was and is a question to which prominence was given in the 'thirties and 'forties by Ruth Benedict, Ralph Linton, Edward Sapir, A. I. Hallowell, and a number of other American anthropologists.[1] There is a good deal of evidence to suggest that some cultures provide roles and patterns of ideas and beliefs in which personalities that we would regard as psychologically aberrant, or even sick, can find legitimate outlet and esteem. The shaman among some Arctic peoples, and similar types of diviners and practitioners of magical and healing arts found in many other parts of the world, are usually cited as examples. The question is how widespread are cultural outlets of this sort and do they indeed take care of all forms of mental abnormality where they are customary? There are also more general considerations relating to what Kiev (1964) calls the 'culture bound' forms of expression of psychopathological states, such as delusions and paranoid fantasies.

[1] Relevant references are conveniently accessible in the bibliography attached to Kiev's paper, 'The study of folk psychiatry', in Kiev (1964).

The Tallensi Notion of Madness

As I have already noted, the Tallensi are innocent of such forms of inspirational divination and healing as shamanism, spirit possession, conjuring, and so forth. Madness, however, is a condition that they clearly recognize by its overt manifestations, and they have a terminology for describing it. The term for a mad person is *galuk*. It implies a state of what we should call craziness. The stereotype of the mad person is that his talk is wild and confused (*gaha-gaha* or *bassa-bassa*) and his behaviour erratic and sometimes violent. He is deemed to be incapable of normal social and personal relationships in marriage, in family life, and in community affairs. He is incapable of taking part in religious and ceremonial activities. Most important of all, and an early sign of the condition, is incapacity to perform normal work, e.g., in the case of a man, the economic activities of farming, or, in the case of a woman, cooking and caring for her children. Furthermore, the Tallensi, like ordinary people in our society, distinguish between madness and other forms of abnormality or eccentricity. Madness is a disease; it has an aetiology and is susceptible of treatment. The others are not regarded as forms of sickness, but rather as congenital, almost accidental, infirmities.

Incidence of Madness

I learnt about these distinctions early in my first period of residence among the Tallensi. Considering how specific they are, it was to me quite tantalizing that in my two and a half years among the Tallensi I came across only one gross case of madness, as judged by their criteria. Knowledgeable people with whom I discussed this case were emphatic in contrasting the condition of this man with that of two other psychologically queer persons known to everybody in the district. One of these, a wizened character who might have been any age between thirty and fifty, might well have been psychotic too. He appeared to have no home of his own and was given to wandering aimlessly about the country. His behaviour was childish but never offensive, and he was generally laughed at good-humouredly. The other was, in my judgement, a high-grade mental defective. His age, at a rough guess, was about twenty-five. He was sometimes described as 'crazy'. But everybody, including his own family, insisted that he was not mad in the strict sense, since he had been this way from birth. He was commonly described as 'lacking sense' or simply as being 'stupid'. Unlike anyone regarded as really mad, he was often upbraided for causing annoyance by his boorish manners and importunities. He lived at home and was capable of working on his father's farm and of looking after the livestock spasmodically. Unlike a madman he never went about naked and could take care of himself. Though his habits were erratic, his gait clumsy, and his speech sometimes wild (but not confused), he had quite a fund of the kind of knowledge and information one could expect in a boy of perhaps nine or ten. He was, of course, not married. The idea that he might even aspire to marry, as he sometimes pretended, was greeted with ridicule.

I knew a number of others, both adults and juveniles of both sexes, who seemed to be of subnormal intelligence or of defective personality, but they played their part in the economic and social life of their families in an apparently normal way and were not regarded as mad. The same attitude was shown towards some old people of whom it was said that they were no longer capable of anything but eating and sleeping and making themselves disagreeable. One sometimes saw such an old man or old woman sitting slumped in a corner muttering to himself or herself and neither taking notice of anything nor being taken notice of.

Lastly, there were several people, of middle age and over, whom their families and neighbours considered to be eccentric by Tallensi standards. One whom I knew well was so regarded because he had never married and, like an old-maidish spinster in our society, attended to his household chores himself. Some said that he was so ugly that no woman would have him, others that he had an uncontrollable temper which put women off. But in every other respect he lived like other men of his age.

It is of interest, incidentally, that both homicide and suicide are extremely rare among the Tallensi. No cases occurred during the time I was with them in the 'thirties and the magistrate previously mentioned stated that none had come to the notice of the police in recent years. Indeed he made rather a point of this, since Tallensi are given to heated argument in disputes. Homicide is traditionally regarded with great horror. If the victim is a kinsman it is a mortal sin against the ancestors and the Earth, sure to be visited with the ultimate supernatural penalty of death, and the extinction of the murderer's whole family. If the victim is a non-kinsman the murder would, in former times, have sparked off a feud. Suicide is not a sin but is thought of with pity and contempt. The stereotype is of a person who, plunged into despair by the death of an only child, stabs himself with a poisoned arrow. This is given out as one reason why a person thus bereaved is never left alone until the first wave of grief has passed. I might add that, by contrast, homicide and suicide, especially the latter, quite often occur among the Southern Ghanaians with whom Field's book is concerned.

I have been speaking in general terms of the Tallensi, but to be strictly accurate my closest contacts were with a group of clans within a two-mile radius of my headquarters at Tongo. It was within this cluster of about 5,000 people that the three cases I have referred to turned up. Even, however, if we take this population as the basis, the conclusion is unavoidable that overt madness, as defined by the Tallensi themselves, was of negligible incidence among them in 1934–37. The picture today is strikingly different. As Dr Mayer will explain in the third section of this paper, she found no fewer than thirteen Tallensi cases of psychosis in 1963. All of these came from the cluster of clans I have just referred to. This finding cannot be correlated with population increase in the area. With natural increase as the only source of population maintenance it is inconceivable that it could have multiplied thirteen-fold in a generation.[1] What was quite startling, from my point of view, is that several of these cases occurred in families which were specially well known to me in 1934–37 and which were basically the same in structure in 1963 as in the earlier period. I knew some of these patients then as young wives or youths or children. Theirs were the families of my best friends and inform-ants, some of whom are still living. Had such cases occurred among them in 1934–37 I could not have missed them. When we discussed this contrast with some of the elders they insisted, most emphatically, that madness was so rare as to be almost unheard of in their youth and that it had become common only in recent

---

[1] The data for an accurate assessment do not exist but my guess, based on the 1960 census, is that, at the very outside, the population in this area may have doubled in the past thirty-nine years. But the *resident* population seems to have remained nearly stationary owing to the increase in emigration, mostly of a short-term character.

years. They blamed this on gin and other vices imported from the South. Such opinions are, of course, no more reliable as evidence in Africa than among ourselves. I quote them only as circumstantial confirmation of my own impressions.

Case Record

Let me now very briefly describe the one indubitably psychotic case I encountered in 1934–37. Aged about twenty-two, and wearing only a tattered loincloth, *Awola* slouched limply and spoke in a monotonous, muffled voice, but gave relatively coherent answers to questions about his illness and his circumstances. He was not living at home but in the house of a friend of his family, who supplied the details of his story. The reason for this was that his father was blind and lived as a dependant with an uncle, and his mother, who deserted the father when *Awola* was a child, was dead. Unable to farm, my patient, if I might dignify him by such a title, generally spent his days begging in the local market.

Describing the onset of his illness in terms that have remained the stereotype until now, he attributed it to an attack by 'evil trees'. Prompted by his friends, he explained that he was not yet fully grown but at the stage of puberty when his testicles had descended and he was having dreams with nocturnal emissions. He was keeping watch over his father's newly sown farm one day. There were many trees around. While resting at midday he fell asleep. He woke up shivering with cold and fear to find a whirlwind sweeping over him. When, later, he set out for home, he could not walk straight. He could not sleep that night and his body ached. This went on for four days. Noticing that he walked erratically and that his body trembled continuously, his father concluded that he was ill and that it was the illness caused by 'bad trees'. Treatment in the standard form of ablutions with, and potations of, an infusion of roots and herbs was tried and failed. Ever since, he had been unable to farm, babbled confusedly in his sleep, and generally felt weak and listless.

During the telling of this story *Awola*'s attention frequently wandered and a vacuous look spread over his face. He demonstrated the song and dance with which he usually tried to amuse people from whom he begged. They were pathetically childish, as the bystanders pointed out. He was generally treated with patience and kindness and never lacked for food. People said he was harmless. Had he been violent he would have been put in fetters.

An obvious comment occurs to me. It seems to me that the form of magical aetiology invoked by the Tallensi to account for madness corresponds symbolically rather well with the status of the madman in the family and social structure. He is not thrown out of the family as happens in some societies, for he still remains a member and must be cared for as such. But he is not a responsible person able to contribute by his work to the family's income and continuity, subject to the normal social and moral sanctions, and accountable for his conduct to the elders and the ancestors. He is human and yet, by reason of his abnormal state of mind, a-human. What could better symbolize his condition than the notion that he is the innocent victim of motiveless malevolence discharged by non-human objects situated outside the realm of normal socio-religious relationships and morality? There is a parallel with infancy, by the way. An infant is, from the Tallensi point of view, not fully human until he has a following sibling.

The Problem of Increasing Psychosis

I come back, in conclusion, to the question of the apparently striking increase in the incidence of psychosis in this community since 1937. Could it be that I simply failed to detect cases that did in fact occur? I doubt this, since sufferers are never hidden from public knowledge. Could it be that conditions of life were so hard thirty years ago that psychotics died off early in their sickness and so did not come to notice? This view is not tenable, for then, as now, food and shelter were always available to a madman even if he was so violent as to require putting 'in log'. Alternatively, it might be that there were, in the past, as many people predisposed to psychosis as there are now, but that the traditional way of life and social organization, at that time hardly affected by the outside world, either were free of the stresses that precipitate psychosis nowadays or effectively cushioned them. Dr Mayer and I can give no conclusive answer to this question. It calls for further research, on a wider and more systematic scale than we were able to attempt. It is hardly to be doubted that there is a connection between the high incidence of psychosis among Tallensi today, as compared with a generation ago, and the changes that have taken place in their conditions of life during recent years. Just what these connections are can only be guessed at on our present data. The feature that stands out is the propensity for breakdowns to occur in circumstances of alienation from the home environment or from the traditional cultural goals and values.

III OBSERVATIONS ON PSYCHOSIS, 1963

Introductory

We had been in the field only a few days when it became apparent that there would be madmen to interview. Mad Tallensi are like madmen anywhere. Only the latent or borderline cases need identification by a psychiatrist or in fact by anyone with special training. Meyer Fortes's supposition that he might not have been able to find them in the 'thirties because he lacked the diagnostic skill was thus shown to be untenable. These were overt cases and they had all been identified as such by their families. Because of the short time at our disposal and because I was handicapped by having to work through an interpreter, I excluded doubtful or borderline cases. During our ten weeks' residence I was able to secure histories on twenty psychotics, thirteen Tallensi and seven from the neighbouring Gorensi tribe living near Zuarungu. The members of this closely related tribe speak more English than do the Tallensi, wear more clothes, drink more local gin, are more likely to have gone to school and to be at least nominal Christians – and they seemed to have considerably more madness. This impression was based on our experience, not on a systematic survey. We had not intended to investigate these people, but they sought us out. In the area around Tongo I only once saw more than one mad person in a single family compound; in the Zuarungu compounds I visited, after I had seen one I was in every case asked to see others; after a short time, since we were more interested in studying the Tallensi, I had to refuse to see any more Gorensi patients. It might be thought that this group, being more Westernized, would be more willing to seek medical help, but this, as we shall see later, was not the case.

Tallensi Attitudes to Madness

In Western society there is at least some evidence to indicate that any purported increase in psychosis is more apparent than real, due in part to better diagnosis and in part to a new willingness to bring the mentally ill to doctors for treatment. The mad aunt who used to be hidden in an attic, the crazy wife who made life a nightmare for Jane Eyre, are now sent to mental hospitals. This twentieth-century notion of psychosis as remediable, and almost respectable, may explain a seeming increase in England or in the United States, but not among the Tallensi. For their attitude is, and has been, one of easy acceptance. The tact that is so necessary in interviewing relatives of psychotics in the West is uncalled for here. Relatives talk willingly and without embarrassment about the madman in their midst. If he is violent, or given to running away, he is usually confined by attachment to a heavy log; but the patient 'in log' is not hidden away out of sight of strangers; on the contrary, he spends much of his time under the large baobab tree which is the centre of family activity. Their attitude towards him seems singularly lacking in conflict. If he hits out, roams, or destroys property they do not like it, but they do not feel he is responsible. Mad talk evokes hearty, but not cruel, amusement. If he gets well there is no need for a 'half-way house'. He merely resumes his normal place in the family.

This tolerant attitude towards mental illness seems to be related to Tallensi theories of aetiology, which, as has been indicated in the previous section, virtually preclude the possibility of feeling guilty because there is madness in the family. In our society, if one's offspring becomes psychotic one has the choice of two opposite or complementary notions of aetiology, both of which are guilt-producing: either one has endowed one's child with a bad heredity, or one has provided him with a bad environment. The sense of guilt lessens as the relationship widens, but it is often perceptible even in cousins. Among the Tallensi, if one's relative goes mad it is bad luck, due for the most part to a bad tree or a bad stone, as has already been noted.

A comment made to me, independently of Professor Fortes's inquiries, refers to this. 'Trees, but not all trees,' said a Priest of the Earth, 'become alive in the night; some are bad trees; if they talk to a person who is passing they can make that person mad.' A bad tree is discovered by its actions. However, it does not always act so straightforwardly; it may be more devious, especially if it covets something of yours: 'The tree may turn itself into some person you know and ask for something . . . if you refuse, it can make you mad . . . it may turn itself into a stranger or even a kinsman.'

Causes of Madness

The idea that madness is caused by witchcraft or sorcery is, as has already been explained, exceptional here. Such ideas are prevalent in the South of Ghana, and Field's descriptions of their ramifications (Field, 1960, p. 38), especially of depressed patients accusing themselves of being witches, are in marked contrast to what is found in the Tallensi situation. In each of my cases I asked the patient and the relatives their opinions as to the cause of the illness. Except by a very few people, all of whom had spent a number of years in the South, neither witchcraft nor sorcery was ever mentioned. In the one instance where witchcraft was brought up it was done hesitantly; and the three or four people who talked of the possibility of sorcery (inflicting injury by the use of poison or bad medicine) did so without great conviction. For example, there was *Nafo*[1] who had been stricken with madness nine years before. Since that time he had done little work and was given to periodic outbursts of self-mutilation. His illness had begun while he was working for a farmer in the South, clearing a field for farming. He thought that among the trees he had chopped down there must have been a bad tree which had then taken revenge on him. Almost as an afterthought he said that it might have been his employer who used bad medicine against him. I then pressed him as to which explanation he thought more likely. He answered: 'If I had stolen from the master he might have done it . . . but I did not steal from him.' His brother agreed emphatically that it was not the employer but a bad tree. In striking contrast to the 'paranoid personality' which has impressed some observers in Southern Ghana (cf. Field, 1960), these people tend to think well of themselves and of others and their expectation of being liked and well treated is very obvious.

Description of Sample

The present study comprises seventeen of the psychotics previously mentioned, thirteen Tallensi and four Gorensi. Three of the seven Gorensi originally seen are not included, two because they refused to be interviewed and one because her psychosis

[1] All names of patients in this paper are fictitious.

seemed to be complicated by mental deficiency. The sample could have been larger had I not excluded the elderly, where there is always the special problem of evaluating the organic component. The Tallensi themselves distinguish the madness which comes on in youth or middle age from that which comes on gradually with increasing years and which is a not uncommon concomitant of old age.

My final sample of seventeen cases is obviously too small for any sort of statistical generalization – except in comparison with Professor Fortes's observations of thirty years ago. It is, however, rather different from samples described in other studies of African psychotics in that each patient was seen in his own home, none had had treatment except of the sort described later, and none had ever been to a mental hospital. (Incidentally, the Tallensi do not have healers' shrines of the kind described by Field, 1960, p. 87.) In each of the cases a history was given to me by a family member, usually by the head of the household assisted by several other relatives. The history was followed by an interview with the patient and usually by several follow-up interviews in his own home over a period of several weeks.

The families of all but two of the Tallensi were known to Professor Fortes and he was therefore able to confirm their assurances that there had been no mental illness in their families thirty years ago.

My final sample comprised eight men and nine women. All were non-literate and only one spoke some 'coast English'. All but two (Nos. 3 and 16 in the *Summary Table*, pp. 68–69), who had spent some years in Southern Ghana and had worked as domestic servants for Europeans, had followed traditional occupations or had worked as unskilled labourers at some time. Only one woman (No. 7 in *Table*) and one man (No. 3, referred to above) professed to be Christians but they no longer participated in church services. Their age range, which can only be approximately stated since non-literate Tallensi do not know their ages, was from about fourteen to about fifty. Duration of illness, at the time of my first interview, varied from one day to ten years. However, all but three might be considered chronic in that their illnesses had lasted a year or longer, the average being about three years.

Forms of Psychosis Observed

I had expected, or at least hoped, to see some forms of psychosis that could not be classified according to Western terminology. That I did not do so may be due to the relatively small population in which we were working, but it is worth noting that Leighton, Lambo, *et al.*, in their epidemiological survey of the Yoruba (1963, p. 109), also failed to find symptom patterns which are not recognizable in Western psychiatry. I looked out for the possibility of neurological disease and, so far as I could tell by crude clinical methods, it was not a factor in any of these cases. I saw one patient who had been treated for trypanosomiasis but it did not, as the history and progress showed, seem to have any bearing on the case.

Two cases were affective. One, the youngest of the group, was clearly manic; she was hyperactive, euphoric, talked incessantly and under great pressure. Her judgement, according to her rather exasperated relatives, was poor, but her reality sense was intact. They seemed to find her more maddening than mad. The other was a depression which could, because of the age of onset, be called an involutional melancholia. She too was almost classical by Western standards. She was the sort of woman one used to see so often half hiding in a corner of a hospital corridor, miserable, self-effacing, and yet almost exhibitionist in the way in which she proclaimed her worthlessness. *Bugre* appeared always with an old tin bucket covering her head. She worked but did not bother to eat unless someone put food in front of her. Leighton *et al.*, in the Yoruba study already referred to, found that Yoruba depressed patients had symptoms similar to those found in patients in the United States except that they did not feel guilt (1963, p. 141). Collomb and Zwingelstein, studying depressed patients in Dakar, found a low proportion of guilt and a high proportion of ideas of persecution (1961, p. 227). As has been previously noted, the Tallensi seem very free of guilt, but *Bugre* certainly looked and sounded guilty as, turning her face away and speaking into her pail, she said, 'Yes, I am unhappy but I can't help it . . . because of me my whole family is unhappy but I can't help it.'

The great majority of my cases (thirteen of the seventeen) were clearly schizophrenic, that is they had illnesses characterized by disturbances in their conception of reality and in their relationships

with other people. Their talk showed a loosening of association and was often unintelligible to others. In only a few cases
were there delusions or ideas of reference but, surprisingly, in
comparison with American schizophrenics, there had been a history of hallucinatory experience in every single case. They all
showed affective and behavioural disturbance of varying degrees
of severity. Two other cases, although showing schizophrenic
symptoms, I have classified separately: one lasted only three days
in all, and has therefore been called an acute psychotic episode; the
other, since it occurred about a month after delivery, has been
called a post-partum psychosis.

In considering the matter of further subdividing the schizophrenics into types, I found some difficulty which was, however,
in no sense different from that which I have always found in such
taxonomy; and the reason, here as elsewhere, is that there is
generally a mixed picture. Crudely classified, according to predominant symptomatology, two were paranoid, one was cata-
tonic, and the rest would fit best into the category of either
hebephrenia or simple schizophrenia.

The low incidence of depression and of paranoia in my small
sample is markedly different from the findings of Field in her work
in Southern Ghana. In a sample of fifty-two chronic schizophrenics
she found that over half of the twenty-six males had paranoid
features and nearly half of the women were depressed (Field,
1960, pp. 450–1). I would assume that this discrepancy reflects
not differences in the points of view of the observers but differences in the cases observed. It underlines the truism that one must
be wary of generalizing even about Ghanaians and certainly about
all Africans.

The Clinical Picture

Aside from proportional differences in kinds of psychosis and in
types of schizophrenia, I did find a few unusual features in the
clinical picture in this area which are, I think, worth noting.
Patients were much more willing to meet and talk with me than
I would have expected, and even those who were very withdrawn
showed little or no hostility towards me. That they were much
more willing than American patients to talk about hallucinatory
experience was probably less surprising and had to do with their
simplicity, in that they did not regard this symptom as a stigma.

Two patients who had refused to say anything before I asked if they had had such experiences suddenly broke into a friendly smile by this demonstration that I had some special understanding of them. As in our society, auditory hallucinations were most common. When I asked what the voices said, nine of the fourteen who had such hallucinations were willing to give me examples and, of these, seven described kindly voices which said such things as 'I like you', 'You are good'. Only one heard the sort of voice that is commonplace among Western psychotics, the voice that calls one bad and insulting names. As Bleuler (1950, p. 97) says, 'Threats and curses form the main and most common content of these "voices".'

Possible Connections with Child-rearing Methods

It is intriguing to speculate as to why Americans or Europeans usually hear bad, jeering voices when they have a schizophrenic breakdown, whereas Tallensi and Gorensi hear kindly voices. Although one can only suggest it as a project for more intensive study, it is tempting to associate this with their indulgent methods of child-rearing. Young Tallensi children live in a world that is beset by very real dangers in the form of accident, illness, and sometimes physical privation; but the people with whom they come in contact seem almost invariably loving and benign.

Professor Fortes has referred to Tallensi child-rearing practices but I should like to say something about how they struck me as a non-anthropological observer.

Most observers of African peoples comment on their loving and benevolent attitude towards babies. Tallensi mothers are no different from other African mothers in carrying their babies about with them (on their hips rather than on their backs), feeding them 'on demand', and leaving them, if this is necessary, in the arms of other equally indulgent women, grannies or co-wives, and later in the care of older, but often not much older, sisters and brothers.

I was struck, however, by some features that seem to be characteristic of the Tallensi. Men, as well as women, are extremely affectionate to babies and small children. It is more usual than not, if a man is sitting at his ease, for him to have a child on his lap. If he is eating, he often shares titbits with one or more children. A diviner, sitting in his hut apparently engrossed in his consultation, is in no way troubled if his five-year-old son suddenly crawls in after him to have a better look at what is going on. He may stop for a moment to put his arm around the child before continuing with his serious proceedings.

It seems that there are parts of Southern Ghana where, when the period of early childhood is over, children are treated with 'harsh disregard . . . and the adored small child has to suffer the trauma of growing up into an object of contempt' (Field, 1960, p. 28).[1] Such a transition from being the most to being the least important has been postulated as a possible reason for persecutory attitudes later on. If this is a reasonable hypothesis, it is worth noting that among the Tallensi, who seem relatively free of persecutory attitudes, transitions are very gradual in childhood, and children are never deprived of care and affection.

Breast-feeding, which is the main source of nourishment for the first two or three years, is not stopped suddenly, and even after it has been replaced by the usual solid diet mothers will continue to offer the breast at times of stress. Sometimes when we entered a homestead small children who had never seen white faces before would look at us in fear and dismay; then they would race to their own mothers and almost invariably the mother would offer her breast. After a few reassuring gulps the child would dare to have a second look at us.

From the earliest days infants are cared for by many 'mothers'. As they achieve some independence from the breast, older brothers or sisters begin to take over as part-time nursemaids. But along with the individual care by mother or mother-substitute, they also have very early, and it seems peculiarly satisfying, relationships with their age mates. One often sees children of less than three years with their arms around each other. That other toddlers can at such an early age be seen as friends rather than as

---

[1] From the point of view of cross-cultural comparison, it is not without significance that Field's cases all came from Akan communities with a matrilineal family system that is in many ways quite opposite in structure to the patrilineal system of the Tallensi. This goes with other contrasts in culture and social organization. What is of particular interest is that there are some striking contrasts in child-rearing customs. The emphasis on toilet-training in the first year of life found in most Akan communities (cf. Kaye, 1962, Ch. VII) is the very opposite of the indulgent Tallensi attitude. The practice found in some Akan communities of punishing a child for disobedience or wrongdoing by means of a red pepper enema would horrify Tallensi.

rivals seems likely to have to do with the long period (about three years as a rule) during which the child is the unrivalled possessor of his own mother, while at the same time he is likely to have many age mates because of the 'sisters and brothers' who have the same father but a different mother, or else are the children of father's brothers who live in the same homestead. It may be a peculiarly felicitous situation to have playmates close in age who, on the one hand, have the special closeness of being family members but of whom, on the other hand, there is no need to be jealous because each one has his own exclusive mother to fall back on in time of need.

I do not mean to imply that there is no jealousy when the next sibling actually comes along. As has been mentioned in the first section of this paper, jealousy of the next younger child is an emotion that is known by the Tallensi and accepted as normal. However, I do suggest that the jealousy is something with which the child is able to cope, partly because he is at an age at which he has achieved some measure of independence from his mother, and partly because he already feels himself part both of the larger family and of his own particular age group. It was striking, in every large family we visited, to see what can best be described as a spontaneous nursery-school group which sometimes played alone, sometimes tagged along after older brothers and sisters, and sometimes dispersed as the little ones sought their own mothers or older siblings. The younger groups, by the way, tend to mix girls and boys indiscriminately whereas those comprising children over about six or seven tend to be made up of only boys or only girls.

This digression on child-rearing has to do with my own search for the answer to two problems that appear related: the seeming lack of overt guilt feeling that one observes among the Tallensi people; and the benign form of hallucinatory experience reported by Tallensi psychotics. It should also be borne in mind that it may not be necessary to project bad feelings because they are already incorporated in tangible 'evil' objects, that is the evil trees and stones, as well as, perhaps, in the punitive aspect of the ancestors.

Onset and Precipitation of Psychosis

Another feature worth mentioning has to do with the onset of psychosis. In every case it was described as acute. This does not mean, of course, that there might not have been mild prodromal symptoms or long-term eccentricities that the Tallensi would not in any case recognize as important; however, had they been so extreme as to prevent a person from working (as one would expect with an insidious onset), this would have been noticed.

I do not wish to make too much of this feature since it might be that my inability to speak the language made it impossible to get a history detailed enough to reveal early signs of illness.

On the matter of precipitating events there were some apparently significant coincidences. Of the whole group of seventeen persons, ten had become psychotic while in the South or very shortly after returning from a first trip to the South. It should be understood that for a resident of the Upper Region of Ghana to go to Southern Ghana is still like going to another country; not only is the way of life and of work completely different, but the prevailing language is a foreign one and Northerners are liable to feel at a loss there if circumstances become difficult.

There was no sex difference in this apparent tendency to become ill in the South rather than at home. However, when I looked at the men and women separately, it was interesting to note how many of the women but none of the men either had had peculiarly unhappy life-histories or had become psychotic after a particular traumatic incident. *Tenga* had become ill immediately after the death of her husband; this occurred in the South so she did not until later have the support of her family and, contrary to usual custom, she did not marry another member of her husband's family although she returned to live with them. There was *Atia* who, after having lost two babies in succession, became mad immediately after the death of her husband in Southern Ghana; this happened before she returned home and she too did not remarry. There was *Baaga* (not in the sample because she was one of the Gorensi women who refused to be interviewed) who became mad the day that her second child turned over a cooking pot and was burned to death before her eyes. *Bugre*, the depressed one, had borne six children five of whom had died, and the sixth lived in the South. *Kurug* had not been able to conceive at all – than which there is no worse tragedy, except to have all your babies die.

Response to Treatment

The other difference from psychosis as I had known it before was the surprising response to treatment. It had not been my intention to attempt any therapy. The very idea seemed absurd to an analytically oriented practitioner who was going to spend a couple of months with people whose language she did not understand. However, since I was known as a doctor it was assumed that when I asked to see mad people it was with the intention of curing them; medicine is very highly esteemed and it seemed only reasonable that they would be given some in return for answering my questions.

The hospital serving this area had a limited supply of Largactil in 25 mg. tablets. The amount I was able to obtain from the hospital[1] was so small that it did not occur to me that it would have other than a placebo effect. Had I known that there would be some dramatic results I would have treated half of even my small sample with aspirin or glucose. As it turned out, I could not tell whether it was the small doses of Largactil or the large doses of suggestion that were effective, but the results were startling. Of fourteen schizophrenics[2] treated, generally for a week and in only two cases for more than eleven days, five went into remission, one was greatly improved, four were improved, four were slightly improved or unchanged. If I exclude the Gorensi who, as has been pointed out, have had a longer exposure than the Tallensi to outside influence, the results are still more striking: four of the ten treated schizophrenics went into remission, one was greatly improved, four were improved, and one was slightly improved. My standards for remission were arbitrary. I called it a remission if the person was working as effectively as before the illness, if I could see no residual symptoms and, most important, if the family considered the patient cured. Of the five who went into remission one was the man who suffered the acute episode; he had different treatment from the others as I happened to have a sample of six sparine tablets (25 mg.); I gave them to him over a three-day period. The other four had been ill for six months, two years, two and a half years, and nine years, respectively.

---

[1] I am greatly indebted to the medical officer then in charge of the Bolgatanga Hospital for the help thus generously given to our research project.
[2] The post-partum psychosis and acute psychotic episode are included.

That these remissions were not cures was evidenced by a follow-up study done six months later by an anthropologist, S. Drucker, who was working in a nearby area. Two of the five patients who had gone into remission were as sick now as before, and one who had been greatly improved was now only slightly improved. One who had been improved was now greatly improved, and another patient (not classified as a schizophrenic) who had been unimproved was now in remission. These two attributed their present good health to the treatment they had received six months earlier! The three Gorensi who were seen on follow-up remained as they had been when I left the area except for one patient who had changed from slightly improved to unimproved.

I think we are justified in making the tentative suggestion that among the Tallensi schizophrenia is a more reversible process than it is in a Western society. This possibility is made more interesting by their own belief, stated in informal talks with older men, that madness was formerly more curable by their traditional methods than it is nowadays.

All of the patients I saw had had native treatment, which is different only in detail from that for other sorts of illness. As described to me, independently of Professor Fortes, the first step in treatment is to consult a diviner, for only he will be able to ascertain the cause of the madness. If, as is usual, a bad tree or stone is found to be the cause, the diviner and the owner of the medicine must go off together to locate it and to discover if possible what it was that the particular tree or stone wanted from its victim.

The rest of the treatment is carried out by the 'doctor'. Before starting, he will say to the patient, 'Tell me clear from your heart, do you have any evil thoughts?'[1] It is said that if the patient hides such thoughts he cannot be cured. The next step is to prepare the medicine. Roots are gathered from various trees because of their magical association with madness; for example, there must be roots from a certain tree which has red fruit because of the redness of a madman's eyes. The roots must all be taken from trees that are known to be bad. Bark must then be taken from both the eastern and western sides of the particular bad tree involved. Six ingredients are gathered, including barks and roots from four

[1] I quote from a description given to me by a well-known owner of medicine for treating madness, who claimed to have achieved many cures in the past.

kinds of tree. These ingredients are divided into two piles, each of which contains half of all six ingredients. One of the piles is burned to cinders and for the next few days, three days for a man and four days for a woman, some of the cinders are added to everything the patient eats. The other pile is put into water and boiled each day for the next three or four days. The patient drinks of the hot infusion and is bathed in it every day. This part of the treatment, the drinking and bathing, which forms part of the treatment for all kinds of illness, is particularly intriguing for it repeats a rite that is practised for both mother and baby at the time of childbirth (see p. 38 above, footnote 1).

At the end of the prescribed period, the roots and bark left in the pot are buried in the home compound. Whatever is left of the cinder medicine is taken, along with specially brewed beer and whatever special food the tree desired, by the 'doctor' and the patient to the bad tree. They must go alone and at night. The patient has had his head shaved. They eat and drink sitting under the tree; what is left of the food is buried under the tree and what is left of the beer is poured over it.

If the agent has been a bad stone rather than a bad tree, the treatment is different in some details.

There is, of course, no way of verifying the impression given to us by a number of the older men that such treatment used to be far more effective than it is now. I cannot say that I am convinced of this. But if it were true it might help to explain why psychosis is more in evidence now than it was a generation and a half ago. And if it were true one could only speculate as to why this is so. Perhaps the social changes described by Professor Fortes have undermined the people's faith in traditional treatments. This would be in keeping with the surprising response of my patients to my treatment, which must surely have had to do with their expectations of miraculous cures from Western medicine. Such expectations naturally follow from having witnessed overnight cures of physical illness by anti-malarials and penicillin.

Illustrative Cases

Although no case is ever an average or a typical one, I have selected that of *Awuni* to illustrate some of the similarities and differences between psychosis among the Tallensi today and the picture I am familiar with in the United States and in England.

Awuni was a young Tallensi living in a compound in Tongo.[1] He was about twenty-five years old. He was the eldest son of his father's first wife, and the eldest of all his father's sons. His father had died seven years earlier. The head of the compound was his father's brother whom he called father. His mother was alive and well. The history was given by his younger brother, assisted by the rest of the family. There was no history of madness in the family. The patient was illiterate, and not a Christian; at home he had been a farmer but a few years ago he went South and found work as a 'sanitary labourer'. The family knew of no precipitating event but one day, two and a half years before, he ran into the house of strangers and acted queerly. The people in this house got in touch with his own family. (It should be pointed out here that when members of a tribe migrate South they usually live and associate with compatriots and, even though most of them are illiterate, news travels fast, often by word of mouth.) When the family heard about his illness *Awuni*'s brother went South to fetch him home. He came along willingly enough and even talked sensibly at first; but when they arrived home 'it gripped him' and he ran off into the bush, not returning for three days. Running into the bush is a common early symptom and nothing worries families so much, partly because of the very real dangers. After his return he behaved very strangely. His talk made no sense; he tore up his clothes; if he saw a chicken he would beat it to death then throw it away. That was why they put him 'in log'. (This is a method of confinement in which one foot is put through a hole in a large log. The log is not too big for the patient to drag about, but it is too heavy for him to go very far.) Sometimes they took him out, but then he found people's clothes and tore them up. Sometimes he ate and sometimes he threw away the food he was given; sometimes he sat talking as if to someone who was not visible to the others. There had been *no period of remission* since he became ill.

His family consulted a diviner and called in one herbalist after another but the treatments were of no avail, even though many fowls and a goat had been sacrificed.

This history, although told in the main by *Awuni*'s brother, was listened to by the assembled family who would break in from

[1] This was a family well known to Professor Fortes during his fieldwork in 1934–37.

time to time to supplement with details. *Awuni* sat among them under the baobab tree, his foot stuck in a log. He was well built but skinny and quite naked; he had the vacant look of the schizophrenic. He said nothing spontaneously, but answered questions, although often in a tangential or ambivalent way. When I introduced myself as a doctor he said, 'Where is the medicine?' When I asked him how he felt he said, 'It's inside . . . in my stomach . . . in my chest.' I asked what had happened to him and he replied, 'It happened in Kumasi.' I asked if he dreamed and he said, 'As I sit and talk to you I get hungry.' I ventured, 'Do you mean you don't like my asking these questions?', and he answered, 'Nevertheless, I want them to be asked.'

My interpreter had a hard time asking about voices in Tallensi; and while all the family tried to understand and to reinterpret to the patient, he suddenly began to giggle: 'Yes, . . . they used to be here . . . but not now . . . not very much . . . yesterday it happened.' His voices were kind. 'Sometimes they say, "You are ill", and I say to them, "Yes, I know I am ill".'

I told him I had medicine that might cure him and that it would take about a week to do so (a limit imposed by the number of pills at my disposal). I started him off on 50 mg. of Largactil a day, increasing the dose to 100 and then decreasing it to 50 and then 25 mg. daily. In all he had a total of 825 mg. of Largactil given over an eleven-day period.

The first interview was on 25 October 1963. On the 27th his family reported improvement. He seemed glad to see me, but this time appeared embarrassed about his nakedness and said, 'Tell them to find me that with which to cover myself.' I told the family this was a good sign and suggested that they take him out of log and get him a loincloth.

Eight days later, on 2 November, he was out of log and doing a little work. He looked anxious, moved uncertainly, and had an infected ulcer on his ankle where he had been logged. It had become apparent that his family either could not afford, or would not buy him, a loincloth so we presented him with a fine one from the local market. He put it on rather clumsily while the family stood around offering excited direction and encouragement. He then came forward and thanked me spontaneously. He still seemed to me to be rather apathetic and withdrawn.

Three days later he was unchanged and I stopped the Largactil.

	Name	Tribe	Sex	Age (approx.)	Former occupation	Duration of illness at time of first interview	Diagnosis
1	Nafo	T	M	40	Farmer	9 years	Schizophrenia, paranoid
2	Awuni	T	M	25	Farmer	2½ years	Schizophrenia
3	Anaba	T	M	25	Farmer, had also been a domestic servant	2 years	Schizophrenia
4	Waafo	T	M	25	Farmer	4 years	Schizophrenia
5	Kugri (brother's son to Waafo (4))	T	M	15	Farm helper	1 year	Schizophrenia
6	Yimbil	T	M	55	Farmer	1 day	Acute psychotic episode
7	Baaga	T	F	30	Housewife	2 years	Schizophrenia
8	Tenga (mother of Anaba (3))	T	F	43	Housewife	10 years	Schizophrenia
9	Adongo	T	F	14	Helping in the home	1 year	Affective psychosis, manic
10	Bang	T	F	50	Housewife and seller of beer	5 years	Schizophrenia, paranoid
11	Kurug	T	F	30	Housewife	3 years	Schizophrenia, catatonic
12	Kologu	T	F	25	Housewife	6 months	Post-partum psychosis
13	Bugre	T	F	50	Housewife	4 years	Depression (involutional)
14	Alaa	G	M	25	Farmer	3 years	Schizophrenia
15	Doko	G	M	25	Farmer	6 months	Schizophrenia
16	Atia	G	F	30	Housewife and former child's nurse	3 years	Schizophrenia
17	Soor	G	F	30	Housewife	9 years	Schizophrenia

[1] Egocentric speech here includes various kinds of disordered speech either of form or of content.

Prominent symptoms	Treatment given	Response to treatment 2-6 weeks	6 months
Delusions, auditory hallucinations self-mutilation	Largactil 525 mg. in 11 days	Greatly improved	Slightly improved
Delusions, auditory hallucinations, bizarre behaviour	Largactil 825 mg. in 11 days	Remission	Unimproved
Auditory hallucinations, somatic delusions, bland affect	Largactil 700 mg. in 7 days	Remission	Unimproved
Apathy, egocentric speech,[1] ? hallucinations	Largactil 425 mg. in 11 days	Improved	Unimproved
Bizarre behaviour, inappropriate affect, ? hallucinations	Largactil 425 mg. in 11 days	Improved	Unimproved
Paranoid delusions, aggression, incoherence	Sparine 150 mg. in 3 days	Remission	Remission
Flattened affect, delusions, auditory hallucinations	Largactil 625 mg. in 7 days	Improved	Not seen
Auditory hallucinations, flattened affect, egocentric speech	None	—	—
Pressured, circumstantial speech, inappropriate affect, hyperactivity	Largactil 350 mg. in 7 days	Unimproved	Remission
Aggressive behaviour, delusions of grandeur, visual and auditory hallucinations	Largactil 2000 mg. in 40 days	Improved	Greatly improved
Mutism, catonic postures, hallucinations	Largactil 350 mg. in 8 days	Slightly improved	Slightly improved
Hallucinations, somatic delusions, egocentric speech	Largactil 375 mg. in 8 days	Remission	Remission
Depressed affect, slow speech, expressions of guilt	Largactil 575 mg. in 10 days	Unimproved	Unimproved
Aggressive behaviour, hallucinations, near mutism	Largactil 525 mg. in 7 days	Unimproved	Not seen
Hallucinations, apathy, mutism	Largactil 575 mg. in 9 days	Slightly improved	Unimproved
Hallucinations, somatic delusions, egocentric speech[1]	Largactil 750 mg. in 15 days	Slightly improved	Slightly improved
Auditory hallucinations, bizarre behaviour, egocentric speech	Largactil 625 mg. in 8 days	Remission	Remission

One week after the medication was stopped he was working regularly, and four weeks after the first visit the family considered him well.

We saw him for the last time five weeks after the first visit. He had gained weight, was working regularly, and had begun to talk of looking for a girl. His family considered him cured and said, 'He is now fit to marry.' He did not want to talk about his former symptoms, but he knew that he had been mad and was confident that he was now cured.

Six months later, when seen by S. Drucker, he was naked and in log. His mother said that he had remained quite well until about a month before when he had got up in the night and tried to break down his own room with a hammer.

The second case is of a young woman who had never been far from home. *Kologu* was a young Tallensi of about twenty-five, the first and only wife of her husband. Her mother and father were alive and well, as were her two younger brothers. Nothing unusual was elicited about her childhood. There was no history of madness in the family.

Kologu lived in her father's house until she was in her late teens. One day she was selling her yams in the local market place when a lorry stopped. 'They just took me by force . . . this Ghambigo . . . after three days I escaped from his house.' This was her description of her first marriage. No child was conceived and she remained in her father's house for a year before being courted by her present husband. She married him three years before and said, 'This time it was not by force.'

The patient was a sturdy, pleasant-looking woman who was stripping leaves from a plant when I came to see her. She was shy but not unfriendly and she cooperated with her husband in giving me a history. Her husband said that she had been entirely well until about a month after the delivery of her first child, some seven months before. One evening, after a visit to her father's house, she started to insist that she must take her baby son back to her father. She then began to 'talk bad' (i.e. foolishly, not making sense). Although she cried a lot and talked in this way, she continued to care for the baby who unfortunately died in its fourth month. She mourned the baby 'as any mother would', but in other ways she remained sick. She complained that her body was weak and refused to grind the millet for their meals. She walked aimlessly about the compound and then would sit in front of her house going through peculiar motions.

Kologu told me that she was troubled by seeing people whom others did not see: 'Something was standing by my head . . . others are making noises . . . they say no bad things . . . sometimes they say, "Come, come", and then I go to the market and buy grain and I divide it with them.' Here her husband interrupted to tell me that she did not really go to market at all but wandered around and then sat down and pretended to apportion grain.

They had not consulted a diviner but had seen a local herbalist. He prescribed fowl droppings which they burned in the fire with various roots. She had followed the 'doctor's' prescription and held her head in the smoke of this fire but it had not helped.

I gave her 50 mg. of Largactil daily for one week. On my return visit, at the end of the week, *Kologu* greeted me in a friendly way and thanked me for making her well. Her husband agreed that she was cured and pointed out with special satisfaction that he no longer had to pay to have his millet ground.

The medication was stopped. I paid another visit to the patient two and a half weeks later. She came out of the house to greet me. She and her husband both assured me that she was quite normal again. She no longer heard voices and her body was no longer weak and 'queer'. However, she volunteered that there were times when she felt as if the sickness was coming back. Asked to describe this feeling, she said, 'I begin to think and think and think,' but added with a little smile, 'but I am able to stop myself.'

I considered this a case of post-partum psychosis with features of simple schizophrenia.

She was visited six months later, in June 1964, by S. Drucker, who found, however, that *Kologu* was away on a visit to her father's house. But her husband said that she had remained well.

CONCLUSION

One must of course be wary about drawing conclusions from a few cases seen over such a short period of time. Such results as we found must be stated tentatively and possible explanations even more tentatively, perhaps as guesses rather than conclusions. It seems, however, from this study that:

1. There is more psychosis in this area than there was thirty years ago.

2. There is evidence that there is more psychosis among persons who have been exposed to the conditions of life in the alien and largely urban environment of South Ghana than among those who have remained in their traditional social environment.

3. Among women, there is often a precipitating event connected with marriage or motherhood and this is especially traumatic when occurring away from home.

4. Schizophrenia among the Tallensi is easily diagnosable by Western criteria, the one striking difference in their symptomatology being the relative benignity of their auditory hallucinations.

5. Schizophrenia, at least when treated in the family setting and with the very real support of the whole family, seems to be a more reversible process than it is in more complex societies.

REFERENCES

BLEULER, E. (1950). *Dementia praecox*. New York: International Universities Press.

COLLOMB, H. & ZWINGELSTEIN, J. (1961). Depressive states in an African community (Dakar). In T. A. Lambo (ed.), *Report of First Pan-African Psychiatric Conference*, Abeokuta, Nigeria.

FIELD, M. J. (1960). *Search for security*. London: Faber & Faber.

FORTES, M. (1936). Culture contact as a dynamic process. *Africa* **9**, 24–55.

—— (1945). *The dynamics of clanship among the Tallensi*. London: Oxford University Press on behalf of the International African Institute.

—— (1949). *The web of kinship among the Tallensi*. London: Oxford University Press on behalf of the International African Institute.

—— (1958). Introduction to J. Goody (ed.), *The developmental cycle in domestic groups*. Cambridge Papers in Social Anthropology No. 1. Cambridge: Cambridge University Press.

—— (1959). *Oedipus and Job in West African religion*. Cambridge: Cambridge University Press.

KAYE, B. (1962). *Bringing up children in Ghana*. London: Allen & Unwin.

KIEV, A. (ed.) (1964). *Magic, faith and healing*. New York: Free Press of Glencoe.

LEIGHTON, A. H., LAMBO, T. A. *et al.* (1963). *Psychiatric disorder among the Yoruba*. New York: Cornell University Press.

PRINCE, R. (1964). Indigenous Yoruba psychiatry. In A. Kiev (ed.), *Magic, faith and healing*. New York: Free Press of Glencoe.

SELIGMAN, C. G. (1929). Temperament, conflict and psychosis in a stone age population. *Brit. J. med. Psychol.* **9**.

—— (1932). Anthropological perspective and psychological theory. *J. roy. anthropol. Inst.* **62**.

4 The School as a Therapeutic Community

G. A. LYWARD

I am anxious that what follows shall not fail to leave it quite clear that throughout fifty-seven years of work I have kept in close and active touch with all branches and aspects of education, and I would ask that no value be attached to my comments if they appear as those of someone who has drawn his conclusions merely from forty years of work with maladjusted adolescents of high or good intelligence.

Perhaps I should be a little biographical. I came to my present work from sixteen years as a schoolmaster, having at one time organized the English department in a day school of six hundred boys and served subsequently as a housemaster and sixth-form master at a public school. Unless my testimonials lie I was not a rebel. The point, however, that I wish to make here is that I came to therapeutic work largely as the result of many years' exploration of how best to teach subjects. The history of that exploration goes back to my university days, but it was not until somewhere around 1925 that it began to dawn upon me that my previous and current success (as a teacher of subjects, I mean) was due to the fact that I was engaged in liberating the pupil as a person.

I used to be surprised at the discussions about laziness, inattention, indifference, and so on that I heard among certain colleagues. Frequently a boy with a reputation for all these showed a lively interest within a group I was teaching. How had this come about? I would not discount the interest inherent in any subject of the school curriculum; nor that my own interest may have been infectious. But there seemed more to it than that and I do remember being asked by a colleague somewhere in the 'twenties what my secret was; I could not tell him.

It had something to do with the 'general atmosphere' that

75

developed within the classroom, created by me but not by me alone
– created by everybody in the room by virtue of his being allowed
to be a person. That remark takes me back as far as 1912 when I
first stood in front of a group of children and the thought came
to me, almost like a blow, 'These are people – we are all people
together in a room – that is the most important fact about this
situation.' That they were my pupils (with emphasis on both
words) was a secondary fact completely dwarfed by the first
almost alarming realization.

I am sure that many nursery school teachers and primary school
teachers would know what that experience meant to me. But how
many other teachers retain, if they ever had, that order of values?
There are in secondary schools teachers who do, but what per-
centage do they constitute of the total number of those who teach?
For how many is it but lip service? (And if there can never be
many, what can be hoped for?)

In 1961 I received a letter and a signed menu card from a group
of men in their fifties sitting together at an old-boys' dinner.
From 2B 1916: 'We wish you to know that we will not forget –
ever – former years. All of us (at the annual dinner) had one thing
in common – a profound respect for your teaching and your
influence on all our lives.' That was very humbling. I quote it
because I am trying to say that there is a link between my teaching of subjects (or the atmosphere within which I taught them –
the derivative place I gave to them) and the therapeutic work in
which I have been engaged during the past forty years. What am I
justified in concluding from that? At the least that I was prepared
from the start to take into account the possible fears, guilt, per-
fectionism, self-pity, and so on that so many of the pupils brought
with them to school from their homes and their earlier lives, and
that affected their approach to the subjects of the curriculum. They
were sometimes unable to believe that mistakes were not minor
crimes, unable to ask questions which might betray weaknesses,
unable to plunge in. There were more subtle problems than these:
actual aspects or points in a subject that baffled or revolted them
for reasons connected with their personal lives. Specific difficulties
in specific subjects turned out to reside not in the subject but to
be related to specific emotional disturbances in the pupil.

I am concerned here with what I have called the total atmosphere; for me in those days it was that of my form-room, later

also of a house; in these days it is the total atmosphere of a therapeutic community of about fifty-five people, forty-five or so of them boys and young men sent as seriously maladjusted.

The way of life which is Finchden Manor has had many encouraging things said about it by numerous visitors. May I quote two of the most recent, because words occur in their letters which I have so far not used. A visitor from Switzerland who stayed a fortnight wrote about

> ' "the living together" in the deepest and truest sense of the words and not in the superficial and materialistic meaning of its use nowadays. I am sure that this is one of the main differences between Finchden Manor and most of the other places, as e.g. hospitals, where there is always an enormous gap between staff and patients . . . [where] the well-defined roles help to build up new and more defences. . . . This lack of rigid structure of your community opens the way to the very heart of each personality and breaks down all the wrong defences. . . .'

A visitor from a university wrote of Finchden Manor that

> 'its outlook and values acknowledge another dimension of life that is often overlooked . . . it is a pity that all the students on our course are not able to come to you for a while. It would be much more worth-while than many of the placements: affecting one's whole understanding of, and relationship with, other people rather than merely extending one's knowledge of how institutions are run.'

I would ask you to remember that those comments were not made by me and that there have been, I think, hundreds in a similar vein.

Note these words and phrases: 'relationship'; 'institutions are run'; 'living together in the deepest and truest sense of the words'; 'enormous gap'; 'lack of rigid structure'; 'another dimension'.

I will take the expression 'how institutions are run' because that brings us straight to the first question I expect to be asked: 'At what point does organization become inevitably important?' 'How unstructured can a group be or remain once its size has passed a certain number?' 'Have you a contribution to make to education as a whole over and above any you may have to make to the group treatment of adolescents who are deemed maladjusted?'

At Finchden Manor we do not have rules and sanctions. I believe I have said somewhere that instead of strict rules we have stern love. This is a possible alternative only where members are disarmed. For those disarmed people can be allowed a latitude that they will rarely abuse. But who, you will say, could disarm every member of a school of a thousand girls and boys? Anyhow, are they armed, most of them?

I think that a very large number of them are. *The Times Educational Supplement* contained a review of the book about Finchden Manor in 1956 and concluded that there were hundreds and thousands of girls and boys in need of 'Mr Lyward's Answer'. Dr James Hemming stated fairly recently that one out of every ten children is rejected by his or her fellows.

And we live in strange new times, times in which, to quote Herbert Agar (*A time for greatness*), 'The world wide attack on civilization is forcing us to choose between a worse evil and a better good than mankind has ever known before.'

The growth of the empire of man over himself does not keep step with the growth of the empire of man over nature. There is tremendous mental exploration and control of matter and alongside it a reduced sense of personal values. These thoughts are widespread and they keep us in mind of the fact that we may well need education which is real nourishment and not the competitive pressure from which our young people suffer. (I could tell you of a school which has day boys as well as boarders and of how the mothers of these day boys talk incessantly about their sons' successes in 'O' levels and the like.)

Nourishment (*educare* means 'to nourish') may well be theirs only in so far as their group life helps them to realize that contract, however much it must be the basis of political and commercial and industrial life, is not the basis of human relationships at all levels. People can very soon become things, objects. They can very soon 'learn' to traffic in friendship, in all the imponderables, to value a gift without awareness of a giver. Mechanization and the abstraction of science – all impersonal – have played their part in reducing the power of sentimental religion and that kind of projected egocentricity which encourages an absolute taking of sides with virtue and a failure to realize that it is possible to be in bondage to that – 'Mummy, why are the good people so horrid?' – fortifying self-centredness.

In the midst of a mechanical age when the religious solution was often seen to be projected egocentricity, it was the psychologists who came forward with their solution to the problems of personal relationships – their solution, an approach in depth, may perhaps now be interpreted as pointing to new kinds of group life.

Unlike sentimentality or dialectic conflict – the 'third solution' would be one in terms of imaginative, enlightened love. It would not leave us helpless as the result of self-conscious man's having been clever enough to split the atom.

I once summarized, in a paper I read about Finchden Manor, its need as follows: 'The energizing discipline of non-contractual living together without labels, formalized sanctions, or superficial fairness makes for play and recognition and for awareness and the genuine "please" and "thank you" that reveal non-face-saving health.' This was not my way of saying 'permissive'.

A well-known historian gave us the phrase 'from status to contract' to describe the change from medieval to modern history. I feel that our young people by the thousand need the kind of group experience that will free them from fear, guilt, and the sense of inferiority induced by early untimely contractual encroachments upon natural rhythms and rates of mental and emotional growth, so that they have status without an itch for status symbols, which are bankrupting. Surely that reflection will touch a responsive chord in all who are disturbed by the international scene as portrayed to us and our young people so continuously.

A psychiatrist who visited Finchden Manor recently wrote about the 'very relaxed attitude and behaviour of the boys and the interest and concern they seemed to have for each other'. A sixth-form boy, on the other hand, told me some years ago that 'everyone in my form is bluffing everyone else'. The psychiatrist added that 'in a period when statistics and "success" rates count for so much the tendency must be to try and alter behaviour rather than let it grow and change through growth'.

Change through growth. I am far from denying that many children do develop emotionally but I wonder whether the time is not overdue for approaching young people in such a way that their schooling does not drive nails in the coffins of possibly the majority, by which I mean does not leave them at the mercy of infantile emotions, advertising, propaganda.

G

I tried earlier to make clear that such an approach would not cause a deterioration in academic work but the reverse. For one thing, the young who are experiencing group life at a deeper level than I believe to be true of far too many schools become concerned with quality rather than quantity, become more relaxed and therefore more able to concentrate and will the means with the end. They are also more cooperative. I have a letter by me in which the writer says of Finchden Manor:

> 'I have never come across such spontaneous enjoyment of work and learning for its own sake anywhere except at Oxford. I hated teaching because I had to teach things people didn't want to learn at a time when they didn't want to learn them . . . but I can see in your methods how wonderfully satisfying teaching can be.'

I may talk later about 'my methods' but the point I want to emphasize is that all our energies at Finchden Manor are directed in the first place to maintaining group life at depth. That depth is vital to its members. It lies behind the sense of security, the initiative, the cooperation, the avoidance of cliques or gangs, the concern for the truly moral – and behind scholarship.

Parents and society press for premature crystallization, for the locking up of children in success and economic security, regardless of the war within and the war without. I suppose civilization would collapse if enlightened self-interest were suddenly to disappear. But as I think of the people (for instance Children's Officers) who have pleaded, without response, for time, tolerance, and greater hospitality to experience, I wonder how far education is free of the charge of actually furthering the opposite danger, to wit, collapse into chaos as we go our clever but self-willed way and moralize our mechanization: paying homage to the cortex, a cutting-tool of later development, further removed from the source; confusing the discrete analytical mind with the mind as measurer.

I am not quarrelling with technology or with any of those things necessary in an industrial society but only with the effects of wrong timing, with the dangers of producing people who are schizoid, people for whom reason is detached from the orb of consciousness so that it becomes ratiocination and is always involved in antinomies.

And where relationships are concerned, I want more people to be able to distinguish between 'knowing' and 'knowing about'. I am concerned with living together, which can span time and space where necessary. 'Knowing about' is important, but where other people are concerned 'knowing' is all-important. Knowing makes it possible to dispense with much that is usually called discipline. So many children suffer to some extent from the effects of a moralistic and legalistic discipline that is lazy. I do feel that the *spirit* of the discipline that I have to maintain as prerequisite for healing is vital to the total education of adolescents, when science can lead astray and humanism cannot release a powerful enough spiritual force to counter the destructiveness of our times; for planners are liable to forget that it is people who will have to maintain their organizations and that the task of education is to help in creating the men and women of elasticity and courage and reverence who will create the new society.

Inner processes take time, growth, and inner consolidation; and over and over again nothing seems to be happening – and nothing can happen if pressure and judgement are maintained as they are by society and by so many parents who cannot abide uncertainty. Spontaneity is lost if young people respond, say, to angry words and fall back on rules of duty, politeness, philanthropy, and so on, missing the living moment. T. E. Hulme said: 'Clarity is not the truth; science is not reality.' Standards applied indiscriminately, deadlines which are not lifelines – these can prevent young people thinking clearly. Let no one imagine that I am not all in favour of clear thinking. A poet once told me that he thought that the spirit of Coleridge hovered over Finchden Manor. Well, it was Coleridge who said: 'It ought to be our never-ceasing effort to make people think, not feel.' To think is to be released from the tyranny of feelings. Heart and head together is the way to fuller life and richer relationships.

Can we distinguish between four kinds of group life? There is the quasi-hotel; then the group that is governed largely by rules and regulations and sanctions; then group life which is involvement; and, lastly, membership one of another.

Freedom is a subject that young people like to discuss. Many of them want to turn the place to which they go into a kind of hotel, where they can come and go at will, without much regard for other people and without having more than a peripheral relation with them. They are not very interested in what I will call centres. They live on the edge. Ironically enough, those who have not referred to a centre are the ones who want a reference later. I would like this word centre to remain mysterious – there is a real place for mystery in human relationships within the group. When I say not this nor that (its apparent opposite) but a third, I am not pinpointing the third.

Peripheral relationships may be exciting in the sense of providing 'kicks' but they do not show much play, movement backwards and forwards – concerning which the mother rocking the child in her arms offers a clue, as do children's games: peep-bo, see-saw, hide and seek. This backward and forward movement, which is virtually weaning, is a way to security, emotional security, and towards a life lived in freedom of spirit. I am not going to dispute the fact that life is a challenge – see-saw is also a preparation for that. But because it is a challenge, we must make sure that the early challenges are made within security. Some of these challenges will actually help to create security, but they must be made to someone who feels that he 'belongs' and that he counts for himself, not because of what he can do or does do or because of what he has done. Conversely, security is a great challenge – because once you loosen the texture of your community life and allow for movement, the patterns begin to quiver and the child or young person is not any longer able to lock himself up in them (except temporarily) or manipulate people and situations in terms of them. Then he is forced to internalize, is unable to escape into his blind or semi-blind pushings outward. He develops a proper sense of self-protection and then creativeness. All this is movement away from diminished responsibility.

Loosening of group life allows true incentives to operate. The word incentive is connected with the word incantation. The teacher's joy is to keep free enough to have time to sound for each member that note which is his note, the one to which he cannot help responding because it is his note. Those teachers whose eyes are on their syllabuses can rarely sound a variety of notes.

And what do they meet with? Resistance. I sometimes wonder why so little attention is paid to the total amount of resistance that must dog and fog the teacher/pupil relationship up and down the country and leave so many young people without experience of true scholarship – once again, I am relating group life to scholarship or loss of scholarship. And I had better interpose here that I do not ignore the number of boys and girls who win scholarships under our present system of education. But my contention is that in a certain kind of group at depth, every member becomes in his own way a scholar capable of communication. Subliminal advertising and artificial insemination – these two can stand as indicating the kind of way in which real communication and communion are being, as it were, cut across so that it is extremely easy for people to be denied creative relations with others while hardly knowing that this is taking place and without themselves being known. This seems to me to be a current problem in cognition and recognition.

The resistance that I have to remain aware of in my work, and would have more teachers aware of, is not what it can appear to be. It is not a refusal to accept specific challenges so much as an inability to change, at the bidding of another, a total emotional condition which has perhaps years of repetitive behaviour behind it. The resistant ones – I nearly said the 'lordly ones' – are like squirrels in a cage. They have been hugging a particular and limited and finally negative set of thoughts and feelings, largely related to self-pity. Self-pity has come to replace true self-love, which manifests itself primarily as self-preservation, and then as self-control, which is part of expansion of consciousness, and as creativity.

Just as it is easy and common to mistake his nuisance value for the child himself, so it is common at a later date to confuse him with an external success, a rapid return to good behaviour, or what could be called the passing of an examination. The human nuisance is then, as it were, liquidated or shut up in this examination success. What if most of those whose reports state that they could do better would do better if there was more recognition of the nature of such resistance as I have tried to outline?

What kind of resistance does the teacher so frequently put up to confuse the pupil? I suggest that it is the rigid standard.

Mothers are accustomed to wean their babies from milk to (say) meat. But other matters, surely they are different? Whereas a child cannot be blamed for not holding a cup at the age of one month, we know that quite little children can be convicted of fibbing and slapped for it and we know that older little children can be threatened or persuaded or seduced into behaving well.

So why not always 'deal' with the child's 'bad' behaviour or the young person's shortcomings in his or her work without more ado? Why leave parents and teachers lost – without standards?

Suppose it is suggested that the 'whole baby' is engaged when he drinks the milk and that it is not always the whole child who is engaged when he is acting bravely or being well behaved or learning French verbs? How much does it matter if a child is honest, well mannered, thoughtful, up to scratch with only one part of himself? What may be happening to the rest of him? This, asked in very untechnical language, is a question to disturb.

Is not the vital question: How far is the child doing what he does with his whole self – his 'heart and mind and soul'? Is his heart in his work and play, is he cooperating in freedom of spirit, is his homework spoiling the quality of his sleep, are his friendships free? Or is there a serious gap between the part of him that is answering a challenge and the rest of him? Is he implicitly asking us to get between him and that fear or seduction that is compelling him to be unreal in his bravery or politeness or success, as he makes a dangerously partial response?

In the olden days of not so long ago, we were not awake to the dangers of the partial response, partly because we knew it sometimes could not be avoided. We were concerned, perhaps, with what neighbours were thinking, with how much trouble the child was causing us, or with a lifeless picture of 'what ought to be'. Some of these and similar concerns are quite important but they are not as important as a person's capacity for learning from life, for tolerating the existence of others, staying the course, 'dying daily'.

A child can give and take only after or while he is being nourished. Some need to take more and for longer than others. Taking will look dishonest or selfish to those who have expected it to cease. Yet the wrong kind of stricture by parent or teacher with a child who is taking may deflect him into taking in still stranger ways, and then he will be labelled and it will take more time while he is restored with the aid of those who are willing and able to stand between him and whatever is compelling him to remain unfulfilled and partial in his response to challenge. As things are, however, he is often being forced to live on credit.

All subjects of the curriculum of a school can minister to the child and his society. It is an irony of my life that I came to healing through a discovery of how to use 'subjects' to release and emotionally re-educate young people, but that now I frequently have to plead or insist that they should be protected from formal subject-teaching so long as it can hold up the emotional liberation of the seriously maladjusted.

I hope I still appear to be talking about the atmosphere in which children and young people can be helped as people in schools – and, I would add, in universities.

When bluff is not needed and there is willingness to say and write what is 'felt and thought' rather than what the teacher wants (or what the university library will tell us about what somebody said about what somebody wrote), there come an alertness and honesty and sensitiveness that make every talk and other activity personal, ensuring that there is no serious and traumatic lack of the experience, 'It dawns on me'.

If one ponders over standards as they are only too frequently applied by teachers one soon finds oneself asking how often a child attacked or criticized for failing to reach a rigid standard has developed or suffered from an increasing sense of insecurity and painful separation. Recall how hard it was to 'make it up' when as a fourteen-year-old you had quarrelled with your friend. Recall the lesson following the quarrel and the teacher who hit out at you for not paying attention. Remember the person who made you completely sure that he would not laugh at you or alarm or over-challenge you when he was teaching you to swim. Contrast him with the person who merely said, 'You can trust me,' but never managed to convince you that you could safely let go. Note how, even now, you can make all the difference to somebody from whom you have had to borrow a £1 note if you say convincingly, 'Now don't be at all shy about reminding me if I forget about it. I really shall not mind.' And, while with the word 'forget', acknowledge how hard many people find it to say simply 'I forgot' instead of 'I was about to . . . but just at that moment . . .'

In my community I must resist attempts to persuade me into trying to make the best of two incompatible worlds, the shallow and the deep group life. I would say, after fifty-seven years' experience, that basic skills develop and cultural and academic advance takes place in a sort of inverse proportion to much that is ordinarily considered essential. I suspect that what I have found to be vital for those who are intelligent but emotionally and socially retarded is not without significance for the so-called normal and those who teach them. I know many teachers who are not content to measure and praise and reward a merely partial response in their pupils. They know that it is only within a group living in depth that the drag of the herd can be recognized for what it is. They know that it is better to make challenges intuitively than with an eye fixed on standards. But the intuition must develop out of the deep level of group life. Academic and other efforts which actually replace membership one of another by contract and sap energy are suspect, however satisfying the immediate results may appear to be to the individual or to the community. Academic advance should as far as possible be an aspect of personal development which enables people to give to the community and makes them (to quote Professor John Danby writing about Finchden Manor) 'capable of being alone – alone with the truth and for the truth's sake'.

Our age needs such people. Neither smatterings of knowledge nor intellectual prowess nor unfocused idealism make inevitably for that 'better good' which Herbert Agar wrote about and to which I referred earlier. Is it possible that what is found to restore the maladjusted would make for the nobility of the so-called normal?

In recent years adolescents have been claiming to be a new race. There is now something of a mythology of adolescence. Headmasters and headmistresses are having to wrestle with problems created by the more rapid physical maturing of their boys and girls.

It might be easy to point only to the destructiveness of the age we live in (the essay I wrote for my degree some fifty years ago was 'We are now entering a new dark age').

Modern man is at his wits' end, beyond exhaustion point. Those who have been brought up during what is probably the end of the Renaissance era will note with piety the decadence. They will find it hard to believe that we may well be at the end of an era – that era which looks back to Greece and Rome. But there are not so many of those people living now and they with their authoritarian attitude clash with those others whose attitude is existential.

At Finchden Manor we try to bring about a melting of these two groups, keeping in mind that, as has been said, 'those who

dogmatize . . . insult the wind as it blows'. Often when I am confronted by a clever sixth-former who has come to grief he will
try at first to defend himself and his 'new race' with such statements as 'What is wrong with self-indulgence?' Then I hope that
I am perhaps surveying not decadence but what I have heard
called 'procreant putrefaction'. Latin law and Aristotelian philosophy seem to be 'out', as is *Homo ethicus*. These young people
seem to be agreeing with Nicholas Berdyaev when he says that
'among the ancients Heraclitus is most close to me'. The art and
literature of this period show affiliations with the pre-Plato period,
which is, I suppose, not strictly European at all, but rather middle-
eastern.

Personalism and modern psychology itself show these same
affiliations. Heraclitus said, 'Travel over every road, you cannot
discover the frontiers of the soul – it has so deep a logos.' He
emphasizes tension as the true norm of existence. That is modern,
surely; but it is also a reverting to the womb of our civilization.
It has been truly said that when instincts are more sure and significant than conscious mind and will we must be in a period of
extinction or rebirth. Reversions to origins more remote than
Plato may bring about a renaissance more radical and rich than
that which is surely now coming to an end.

What I have just said and that which immediately follows was
first conveyed to me twenty years ago (in a Burning Glass Pam-
phlet – Chaning-Pearce) but came to mean more when I began
to meet beatniks and found myself being patient with them, be-
lieving that it is not loving nor wise to throw out the baby with
the bath water. Their attitudes may be 'rooted in blood rather than
brain, of the spirit rather than of the intellect, mystical rather than
moral'. All this is foreign to my own upbringing, but I am one of
those who have been compelled to accept these young people who
claim to be a new race, knowing that I cannot hope to be accepted
by them if I shut myself off from their hunger for relationships
such as they claim (with varying degrees of conviction) to have
experienced; relationships that are often puzzling but certainly
not always wholly despicable. They are out of sympathy with the
typical European Renaissance man who set out to master the
world. These young people are having to come to terms with
death, the death of the age that we older people only very tentatively questioned, as well as with the bomb. They go undefended

by dogmas and they are self-pitying or creative according to whether they experience shallow group life or group life in depth.

Is it possible that, with some more continuous recognition that children (so-called because of their physical immaturity) are human beings in their own right, facing their own destiny and unfolding their soul-inheritance within the limits of the psycho-physical vehicle the parents have partly provided, a new and wiser attitude towards the younger generation might arise? Wisdom is not merely intellectual acuteness – it includes reverence and sympathy and a recognition of those limitations that bound all human endeavour.

I hesitate, more than I may seem to do, to reiterate the point I am making today, namely that perhaps our educational system is out-of-date in this nuclear age. Granted that we need scientists – we must nevertheless keep in mind that the laboratory-trained are peculiarly liable at present to be cut off from the world of subjective values, thereby preferring large-scale enterprise to small-scale, and falling through panic into totalitarianism of one kind or another. How easily we can forget that our highest most creative moments are those of feeling and direct knowledge.

We should teach to the feeling for the sake of thinking, for the sake of the subject, and still more for the sake of the child. It is only what he makes his own that helps him to think clearly; to live not possessively. To make it his own he must see, synthesize, and seek and find unity. He must not merely analyse or accumulate and so lose gradually the power of keeping alive to the 'mysterious, threatening soul-searching realm of being which lies behind and within the sphere in which organization achieves its ends' – not now in 1969 – or social reform, for example, will express his personal entanglements and be carried out largely in fantasy.

May I now return briefly to the question of teaching technique? It should not be too consistently sequential or linear. Preparation, or 'prep', as it is called, should be preparation (preferably with the teacher) that whets the pupils' appetites so that they can come to the next lesson eager to discover the answer, the solution, the question that emerges from previous answers. There must be play, a certain looseness. What a number of boys and girls have told me how they have been bored by the man or woman who walks round the room dictating history notes and how they have been fatigued.

Seeing, with the eye or inner eye, must take precedence over 'think, think boy, think' (I hope I have made it clear that I am not disparaging thought). Man refuses nowadays 'to trust his eyes, to rely on his senses or to allow what he sees to loosen the bonds that confine his spirit' (Osbert Sitwell, *Noble essences*). Do you remember Robert Bridges in his 'Testament of beauty':

> *... and that the poet guarded this*
> *showeth in his lyric, where of Sylvia 'tis enquired*
> *why all the swains commend her, and he replyeth thereto*
> *Holy fair and wise is she, thus giving to Soul*
> *first place, thereafter to Body and last of the trine*
> *Intelligence: and thatt is their right order in Love.*

These reflections on teaching are relevant to any attempt to plead for group life at greater depth. They are themselves a plea for an unfearful, more leisurely atmosphere, which can keep together all those who are physically together in a classroom. The same adults who appreciate this will be concerned with ethics but will not forget that 'ethics are a means to the attainment of an end which surpasses them'. They will not believe that eight 'O' levels will inevitably protect anybody from the poisons that as a society we administer through our mass media to the most precious part of it, or at any rate the most tender part of it, those who because they are so eager are most easily seduced. They will recognize the danger of perpetuating an unreal 'tradition of fair play which sustains a false idea of social justice and accredits the boy with a slave's mentality craving equality under the tyranny'. Those words were said about schools by a distinguished philosopher writing about Finchden Manor. He added that at Finchden Manor 'the boys learned to trust the staff personally and actively instead of lazily relying on a set of uniform and calculable reactions'.

The welfare state, welcome as it is, presents its problems. We may enjoy a sharing but be in danger, to quote Laurence Hyde, of developing a race of 'under-individualized people sharing inferior experience'.

We cannot and should not wish to turn back the clock. But our schools could go much further than they do in ensuring that depth of group life which would make for lasting creative experience.

I recall that the late Dr G. H. Stead, a wise and much-loved Director of Education, wrote of the 1944 Education Act that it might turn out to be 'in effect an excellent structure but one which might fail in its ultimate content'.

An American experiment in thirty schools contemplated the urbanization, specialization, and standardization that are changing the world which once 'was waiting outside every child's front door'. The experiment aimed to help children 'to cultivate a happy and effective home life, to choose friends wisely and to cooperate cheerfully in worth-while group activities'; 'to face squarely the problems that arise in everyday living and to work out their solutions with an intellectual and emotional balance'; and 'to develop increasing ability to make choices in the light of consequences'.

This involves concentration. Concentration depends upon relaxation. Both are vital to education for leisure – automation is on the way. Neither those whom the French would call *têtu* (many the result of our considering adolescence as primarily a thinking rather than a feeling period of life) nor those whose only hope for their leisure is bingo are ready for more leisure.

The fourteen-year-old school-leaver used to enter the industrial world suggestible rather than teachable (teachableness is the real goal schools should have for their members) and either identified himself with it, losing his play as he became an industrial personality, or became a machine and constructed for himself as compensation a pleasure world which was just as mechanical; or he made of 'service' a refuge from life. What will our sixteen-year-olds do with their leisure?

I should like to conclude with a reference to what I call 'the third', not this nor that but a third, holding together the two apparent opposites as contraries. This third must remain unnamed in so far as it belongs to a new dimension. Its reality constitutes depth in group life and all that derives from it. I was pondering over the possible words that might hint at what is so difficult to convey. I found the following summing-up by myself of a discussion (at London University Institute of Education) between those who taught maladjusted children in day schools:

' "Without the added strain of removal from home" – that is the sentence that has lingered in my mind. The disturbed children about whose rehabilitation we were hearing had had strains and had then been removed from those strains for "easing". The attempt to ease might involve strain.

To envisage "strain-easing-strain" was to recognize a third possibility hidden within the second. This kind of recognition marked the talks. . . . This is the kind of thinking which the heart finds easy. It is born of love rather than of logic. Is it possible that only those who accept the statement "the key to all deeper insight into human behaviour is not technical proficiency but simply love" can know what is meant by "depth of group life" and "deep relationships"?

The speakers were describing atmospheres in which child and adolescent were not above all subjected to rules and regulations nor to a certain kind of linear teaching. This latter can easily assist a child to be not "all there" and because it lacks depth can play no small part in producing a schizoid generation.

As so often nowadays, I found myself pondering upon how the needs of the disturbed child and the approach to him reveal the inadequate nature of so much so-called education elsewhere.

When the study of subjects does not take place within a group life of depth, allowing deep relationships (reducing bluff, bluster, face-saving, and snobberies to a minimum), then there is a danger of young people suffering from what is now a possible plea in the courts, namely "diminished responsibility". These can often see what they are doing as clearly as – shall I say you or I? – but it is as if somebody else was doing it. Their seeing is not effective to give them a sense of self-preservation and a freedom from punishing consequences, let alone freedom for satisfying the demands of a deeper self. They can hardly fail to produce strife or bring into existence a laborious organization which has to try to bring about from without what should develop from within.

Likewise they can, some of them, win scholarships but they are not true scholars. Every child can be that; it is not a question of quantity.

The "quiet presence" of the teacher; non-rejection of the child as he is; freedom to experiment; these play their part in producing an atmosphere of relaxation in which one-time frustrations become challenges such as are welcomed by living *people*. People *living* together are indeed "joyned with an holy boond", as Professor L. C. Knights, quoting Chaucer's Boethius, points out. And we should agree with the comment he makes in his lecture on Shakespeare and Politics: "The love that is in question is not of course simply a matter of feelings; it includes a neighbourly tolerance of differences and a sense of mutual need; and in its openness to life, its willingness to *listen*, it is allied to that justice which gives each man his due, looking towards what he is or can become; and there is delight super-added." '

Power relations, however disguised, are not enough. Richard Church, after a chance encounter with a child, writes of 'candour which makes the world go round and gives the lie to all that Machiavellian protocol through which the human race pursues too much of its social and political articulations'.

© G. A. Lyward, 1969

5 Managers, Men, and the Art of Listening

R. W. REVANS

Several years ago we decided, at Manchester College of Science and Technology, to study some of the factors that steer the cutting-edge of technological achievement, particularly the attitudes of workpeople towards innovation. We felt that it would be helpful to know more of the difficulties that accompany the introduction of new methods, to understand the alarums of redundancy they raise or the contradictions their rewards create; we should also learn more of that opposition to change, rooted not in fear of unemployment or of exploitation, but in the fact of change itself, and should give our examination all the numerical validity our methods would permit.

As a start we invited a number of Manchester firms to let us interview a random sample of their workpeople. The interviews were carried out by a Pakistani mechanical engineer, with wide factory experience, sent to us by his government to learn something of the problems of our industrial culture. Mr Hussain saw altogether about 800 workpeople, men and women, piece-workers, day-wage men, shop stewards, foremen, and managers. His first 500 interviews, some of which lasted three hours, were unstructured; he merely explained where he was from and that he wanted to know what Lancashire workers felt about their tasks; he mentioned especially the effects of work study, since it was through this that many British factories would attempt to innovate. For this reason it was a subject in which the developing nations had a particular interest.

From the records of these 500 interviews, upwards of 10,000 discrete statements were identified; they included facts, rumours, anecdotes, moral precepts, myths, wishful thinking, wild exaggeration, and sheer nonsense. But whatever the content of the statements, it was found that the majority could be classified under one or more of thirty-four separate headings. One such topic was the gearing of wage to output: 'Here we get as much out of work study as the management'; 'The men do all the work and the management get all the profits'; 'The extra you get paid isn't worth the effort you have to make to get it'; 'Although we argue a lot with the boss about our money, we have to admit he's fair in the end'; 'What I like about this place is that you can go for a bit extra any week you want it'; 'Here they make your money up to what you would have got if things hadn't gone wrong'; and so forth.

Other headings were: fears of redundancy ('Work study today; labour exchange tomorrow'); the accuracy of measured times; the alertness of foremen; managerial attitudes to the trade union; pressures from above to work harder; working conditions; suggestion schemes; the disposition of managers to listen to complaints, or even to listen at all. Once the topics had been subjectively identified, the problem then was to suggest their interrelations and their relative importance. Our task was to assess a sample of opinions numerically; merely to list them would be like writing out a medical prescription that omits the quantities of the drugs to be made up.

This evaluation was done in a second study using the results of the first sample. From each of the thirty-four headings a typical statement was selected, one that seemed strongly to illustrate the essential topic. For example: 'If you tell the foreman, he will soon do something about your trouble.' This suggests the general heading of the alertness of supervisors. From the same box one could also draw: 'You can talk to the foreman until you are blue in the face and he still does nothing about the mess you are all in.' But whichever is chosen, the positive or the negative, it can be printed along with thirty-three others, so that all categories are represented on a particular form.

Several varieties of these were prepared, using different statements from particular boxes. These forms were then scored, in confidence and anonymity, by random samples of workpeople, at five levels of response: strong agreement, tendency to agreement, uncertainty, tendency to disagreement, and strong disagreement. Agreement with positive statements or disagreement with negative statements scored positive marks, and vice versa;

uncertainty scored zero; strong opinions scored double. Hence each worker returned a series of 34 marks, varying from +2 to −2. In this second stage, 266 workers from seven different factories responded to statements drawn from the thirty-four headings, giving a table of 266 × 34 scores. This was factor-analysed and showed three main families of opinion: ten of the thirty-four items, strung out in columns of 266 entries, sufficiently resembled each other to be grouped as one family; so also did a group of six others, and a third group of four.

The first group we describe as loaded with the same factor, and we call this (after that one of the thirty-four items most strongly loaded with it) the attentiveness factor. We find that the one item in the consciousness of the workpeople most related to all thirty-three others is their confidence in the capacity of their management to listen to them. The group of ten items, of which this is the archetype, are, as perceived by the workers:

1. Management's capacity to listen
2. Management's essential fairness beneath its manifest toughness
3. Supervision's alertness to operational snags
4. Management's promptness with complaints
5. Gearing of wages to output
6. Division of benefits between managers and men
7. Effort needed to learn a new task
8. Delay involved in changing between tasks
9. Respect shown for individual skills
10. Likelihood of redundancy.

The first four describe (and can be used to measure) attitudes to management. The next six describe (and can likewise be used to measure) certain important attitudes towards working conditions and their rewards, including restrictive practices.

Workers with positive scores towards one of these ten are significantly likely to have positive scores to any of the other nine, and vice versa. A man who, for example, believes that his management does not listen to him tends to fear redundancy; a man who thinks that his supervisor pays no attention to his operating troubles is dissatisfied about his rate of pay; one who, on the other hand, sees his complaints quickly dealt with does not

H

fear that his skill is discounted, feels that he is not exploited by
the management, and is not afraid to go to a new task.

It is useful to express the total scores on the two sub-sets of
items as in *Table 1* below. All we need do is add together the four
scores of items 1 to 4 (with totals ranging from +8 to −8) for
all 266 respondents and also the scores of items 5 to 10 (ranging
from +12 to −12); we then classify each of the 266 by his or her
two scores. We may replace numerical scores by 'human' attributes to illustrate the relationship in familiar terms; if a man, on
items 1 to 4, scores +5 or more, he sees his management as forthcoming; if −5 or less, as hostile; if, on the other six items, his
score is +6 or above, he sees his working conditions as highly
satisfactory, and so forth.

Table 1   Impression of management related to level
of work-satisfaction, for 266 workpeople

Impression of management	Attitude to employment			
	Highly satisfactory	Satisfactory	Unsatisfactory	Highly unsatisfactory
Forthcoming	29	9	2	1
Aware	11	67	10	2
Indifferent	5	6	73	10
Hostile	0	3	14	24

The second group of items suggests a factor of managerial
pressure and the men's response to it: 'No matter how much you
get done, they keep on driving you', etc. These perceptions of
pressure correlate strongly with opinions about the fairness of
work measurement, the consistency of wage-rates, and the inherent interest of streamlined tasks. Men who do not feel under
unreasonable pressure, who are satisfied with the services – like
maintenance and supply – that enable them to work fast, and
whose management, as they see it, works with them as a production team, are prepared to accept the stop watch, do not worry
about pay anomalies thrown up by new methods, and do not fear
that working efficiency means boredom or the depersonalization
of skill. The converse of these relations is again true. The results
are shown in *Table 2*.

Table 2   Impression of managerial pressure related to attitude towards change of methods, for 266 workpeople

Perception of management pressure	Attitude towards improving efficiency			
	Sympathetic	Yielding	Reluctant	Antagonistic
Accommodating	18	6	7	2
Steady	7	81	9	8
Exacting	8	21	70	2
Merciless	0	2	8	17

The third factor that emerges from the analysis is that of human resources: men who see their managements both as respecting the trade union as a positive force in securing change and as seeking the ideas of individual workers do not fear new methods and do not see work study as a threat to older men.

The first conclusions from this study are thus that negative attitudes towards innovation are very significantly associated with the image presented by management. Above all, managements that impress their men with a capacity to listen are rewarded by their men showing satisfaction with their conditions of employment, and managements that do not appear to drive their men at the point of work find them willing to adopt new methods of work.

Nor is this all. We can analyse the responses so as to throw up the differences, not only between the 266 workers, but also between the seven factories in which they are employed. We find two interesting results from this:

1. Factories in which the workpeople as a whole feel that their management listens show throughout satisfaction with working conditions, and vice versa.

2. The differences in these respects *between* factories are over five times as great as the differences *within* factories.

The first of these might have been expected from the first table, but it does not necessarily follow. However this may be, the effect is very significant: the men throughout a whole factory show a unanimity of view both of their management's capacity to listen and of their own satisfaction with working conditions. The quickest way to depress morale is for management not to listen to what the men have to say; the most effective way of arousing hostility to change is to exercise an unyielding pressure; the fear of redundancy is most quickly excited by introducing new methods without seeking union support or individual suggestions.

The second result may be amplified: if we accept that any human beings must necessarily differ in the extent to which they feel their superiors are disposed to listen to them, and if we then set up a measure of this difference among Lancashire workpeople, we find that the differences on this same measure *between* factories are five times as great as those among the human beings *within* any one factory. This means that group factors, colouring the outlook of all in one given factory differently from the outlook of all in another, are five times as important as the inevitable personal differences that distinguish one individual from another. We may not be able to change human nature to any great degree; we hardly need to, since we can get five times the pay-off by changing the climate of the factories themselves – the first table suggests the means of doing so.

Our task is to help managers to learn the art of listening. How is this to be done? For managers, like all other men, learn only what they want to learn, and nobody wants to learn until he admits his need to do so. What, to be realistic, are the possibilities of persuading British managers that their first need may be to learn to listen to what is said to them?

© R. W. Revans, 1969

6 Some Methodological Notes on a Hospital Study

ISABEL E. P. MENZIES

THE SOCIOTHERAPEUTIC APPROACH

This paper selects for comment some aspects of a particular research method and gives as illustration a brief account of a study in a hospital. The research method may be called sociotherapeutic or 'clinical'. The research serves towards the solution of a practical ongoing problem that a social organization is attempting to tackle. It is primarily aimed, therefore, at elucidating the nature of the problem and seeking information on the basis of which the organization may reach a better solution. The main objective of the research is therapy. The research worker's dominant role is as therapist or consultant to the organization. However, it has frequently been the experience of consultants that such studies also produce research findings of a more general nature, which are of practical and theoretical interest beyond the narrow boundaries of the client organization.

Although there are wide variations in the detail of such sociotherapeutic studies, those with which the author has been most closely concerned have tended to follow roughly the same general pattern. The study tends to be initiated by the client organization when one or more of the management affected by the problem make contact with a potential consultant to inquire about the possibilities of getting some help. Before the decision is made to carry out the work, there is a period of initial exploration with a number of objectives:

1. The consultant and the client organization try together to clarify the problem. The consultant will also clarify with the client what research and therapeutic methods are available and may be used. This enables the client organization and the

99

consultant to decide together whether the problem presented is one with which the consultant can help and whether the methods of working are acceptable to the client organization.

2. The initial contacts enable the client organization and the consultant to explore each other as personalities, with their own particular orientations to the problems of social organizations. This is an important exploration, since sociotherapeutic studies of this kind usually involve lengthy and intimate contact between the client organization and the consultant. Any serious incompatibility on the personal level might well jeopardize the work.

3. The client organization and the consultant must mutually explore practical problems such as possible time commitment on both sides, the amount and nature of the work both will be required to undertake, and costs and sources of finance.

If these mutual explorations lead to a decision to work together on the problem, the work proceeds as a variable mixture of research and therapy. Although theoretically separable, research and therapy are likely to be constantly mingled in various degrees at different stages of the study. In the earlier stages, emphasis is likely to be on the research side, in the later stages on the therapeutic side.

The emphasis on research in the early stages of the work can perhaps be more properly described as an attempt to define more accurately the nature of the 'dis-ease' of the organization and to arrive at a more refined diagnosis. The problem that precipitated the approach for help would tend to be treated as a 'presenting problem' rather analogous to a presenting symptom. It may reflect merely the area of the organization's functioning where the 'pain' is most severely felt or can be most easily formulated. Or it may be used as a 'displacement area' because the real disorder is felt to be too close to the core of the organization's being to be easily disclosed either to the self or to others. It is also important to get to know as much as possible about the social organization that is host to the dis-ease.

The need to make a proper diagnosis is as essential in social as in individual therapy. Failure to achieve effective diagnosis might well jeopardize attempts at therapy. There is usually little to be gained by treating a social symptom in isolation: indeed, it may even be harmful. Unless one is reasonably well informed of the real nature of the organization, its dis-ease and its total functioning, there is a danger that one may devise solutions to the presenting problem whose main achievement is the precipitation of other serious problems in other parts of the organization. It is useful to be in a position both to predict and to control the total effects of possible solutions.

In carrying out the more diagnostic or research phase of the work, the main objective is to range as widely as possible with the people concerned around the topics of the general structure and functioning of the organization, its culture, its traditions, its conventions, its formal and informal communication systems, the practical and emotional experiences of its members, the rewards and problems it presents to its members, the formal and informal elements of the interpersonal relationships, formal and informal authority systems, and so on. All is grist to the mill of achieving understanding of the organization and of the presenting problem in its organizational setting.

Because of the width of the canvas, techniques such as highly structured questionnaires do not usually seem particularly appropriate. Unstructured intensive interviews, either with single individuals or with groups, have generally been found more useful. Individuals may be either 'key informants', such as people in key management positions, or individuals selected to represent significant categories of people involved in the problem, e.g. a random 10 per cent sample of all the workers in a certain department. Similarly, the groups may be made up of functioning groups in the organization, or of individuals selected to represent important categories. The aim of the group discussions and interviews is to achieve as free and undirected communication from the informants as possible, and to subject their communications to as little influence as possible from any views or preconceptions the consultant has about the organization, its members, structure, functioning, and problems. At first, at any rate, the consultant has no specific questions in mind that he wants answered. He wants only to learn as much as possible about the organization. This is, of course, a very different research approach from one that sets out to study defined aspects of a defined topic and uses questions prepared in advance.

It is in the group discussions that structure and interviewer/ informant interaction may be reduced to their absolute minimum, and for this reason a diagnostic survey is always initiated with group discussions when the field conditions make this possible. Careful briefing of such groups makes it possible to establish a quasi-free-associative process of communication and of inter- action between group members. To this end the consultant briefs the groups somewhat as follows. The consultant introduces him- self and any colleagues to the group and reminds the group of the present problem, but he also tells the group members that he does not wish them to confine themselves to that topic, and that he is interested to hear about anything that seems to them signifi- cant and important in terms of their own experience as members of the organization. A few very general leads are given as to topics that might be raised. The group members are then asked to hold a discussion among themselves and let the consultants listen to it. A senior consultant sits with the group, ready to intervene if the group gets into any difficulty and needs help, but mainly just listening and observing. A junior colleague records significant aspects of the discussion and behaviour of the group.

Such group discussions have a number of advantages in addi- tion to that of minimizing consultant guidance to communication. They give freer access to personal and institutional unconscious fantasy systems than do other easily usable techniques, because of the quasi-free-associative element. Alternative ways of getting such access to unconscious fantasy systems, e.g. by means of individual projective techniques like Rorschach or thematic apper- ception tests, seem to us inappropriate both because of their clinical pathological overtones and because they are individually oriented whereas the consultant's 'patient' is the organization. However, delineating the unconscious fantasy systems on an institutional basis seems very important. One's understanding of a social organization, as of a person, is likely to be seriously limited if one cannot gain access to unconscious or implicit ele- ments as well as to the more overt ones.

Further, one can often find in such groups a miniature version of the total organization. One can, for instance, watch patterns of interaction between members, which reflect patterns in the total organization. One can observe modes of behaviour, speech, and thought habitual among members of the organization, which

would show less clearly in one-to-one interaction with an out-
sider. By these means, again, development of understanding of
the organization may be greatly facilitated.

The group discussions are not, therefore, used for fact-finding
in the ordinary sense of the word: that is, for providing, or for
providing only, so-called objective facts, overt easily verifiable
data, e.g. about the formal hierarchical structure of the organization, or data that would lend themselves to statistical analysis.
They are used rather to enable the consultant to build up an
account of the 'patterning' of the organization, its structure and
its functioning, its culture, tradition, and conventions, the occupational and personal experiences of its members in both conscious
and unconscious terms. The result is a dynamic account of the
nature of a social system rather than a statement of facts; not only
what goes on, but how, and above all why, it goes on; 'depth
anthropology' would not be a bad description of this operation.

The group discussions also serve as a useful background to the
individual interviews, which must inevitably involve more in-
formant/interviewer interaction and more interviewer-based
structure, however much one may try to develop an interview
out of the leads given by the informant. The group data give some
knowledge of significant areas to be explored and probed more
intensively in the individual interviews, and thus the interviewer
has some assurance that the structure and topics he introduces are
relevant to the study and likely to be so to the informant. However, the individual interviews are also informant-directed to a
considerable extent. It is not important that an informant should
cover all aspects of a topic, since we are not interested in statistical analysis, nor is it important that informants confine themselves to topics regarded now as significant by the consultant. The
interviews facilitate checking, elaboration, and refinement of the
dynamic picture of the organization that has begun to emerge from
the group discussions.

In working with both groups and individuals, the consultant
gives certain guarantees in advance about his professional behaviour. He undertakes to report nothing outside the interviewing
situation except anonymously and to maintain absolute confidence
about any information if the informant so wishes. Such guarantees
place restraints on the consultant which may be somewhat hamper-
ing. The comments of certain informants cannot be anonymous,

e.g. some remarks could be made only by the managing director and would be immediately recognized as coming from him. It is burdensome and frustrating to have information one cannot use explicitly. However, it is our feeling that such behaviour is essential if one is to gain and hold the trust of the people concerned. It is doubtful if much reliance is placed on such guarantees early in a study, but the opportunity to test the sincerity of the guarantees against the consultant's behaviour over time, if he honours the guarantees, builds up trust. This in turn encourages the frankness and sincerity of informants. The data so given are available for the development of the consultant's own understanding, even if they cannot be directly disclosed to members of the client organization.

I should like to make a number of comments on the use of such research techniques before going on to describe other aspects of consultancy studies:

1. I should like to take up further the question of the professional behaviour and ethics of the consultant. By intent, the consultant creates a research situation that aims at making it possible for informants to discuss with him intimate and personal aspects of their experiences in the organization and at allowing the consultant to penetrate deeply into these experiences with them. From the nature of the work, many of the topics discussed are painful and evoke emotional disturbance in informants. The consultant has a professional responsibility to try to anticipate such disturbances and prevent or minimize them, and to deal with disturbances therapeutically when they develop. The possibility of such disturbance is one reason why a consultant cannot necessarily cover all aspects of a topic with all informants. Some areas may be too painful for certain informants easily to expose in a relationship which is basically fact-finding and not therapeutic for them, and where the consultant does not, therefore, have the therapeutic sanction to cause pain. It is important that consultants should have enough intuitive understanding and the necessary experience to be able to assess such situations and work them through reasonably well with informants.

2. The process of analysing and interpreting the data collected by these methods is a complex one and has many potential diffi-

culties. The data do not lend themselves to the use of statistical techniques, or to related techniques for testing validity and reliability. Reaching conclusions depends rather on the clinical and sociological acumen of the consultant and on the soundness of the psychological and organizational theories he uses as a background to analysis and interpretation. Ultimate conviction as to reliability and validity depends on a many-times repeated process of establishing hypotheses and returning to concrete situations in the organization to test and retest them and to refine and elaborate them. Ultimate assurance of their validity depends also on the final test of whether action based on the findings in fact leads to a more effective solution of the organization's problems.

3. In communicating the diagnostic findings to the client organization, one finds oneself in a situation similar to that of the psychotherapist. The clinical data permit of a variety of interpretations, all of which may represent correct insights into the problem. The consultant, like the psychotherapist, has to select which interpretation should be communicated to the client, at what time and in what circumstances, in order to maximize the therapeutic effectiveness of the client/consultant relationship. Many of the data collected may never be communicated to the client, or indeed to anyone else, although they may have been helpful in increasing the consultant's understanding.

A point is reached in the diagnostic phase when the consultant decides that he has enough data and enough understanding of the organization to move with the client into the more therapeutic phase of the study. He will then begin to report back the diagnostic findings and explore their implications with the client. Decisions need to be made now about the form reporting back should take and to whom the reporting will be done. The main choice about the form of reporting is between written and verbal reports. My own preference is for verbal reporting, at least initially, if the situation makes this possible, and perhaps a written report later for reference purposes. The preference for verbal reporting stems from the nature of the therapeutic process. In conveying the results of the study to the client and exploring their implications, one inevitably comes up against resistance to their acceptance which must be dealt with if effective action is to be achieved. It has been our experience that this can best be done in a face-to-face situation when the client and the consultant share the data, explore them together, and face the resistances as they come up. This is an important situation also for continuing the testing, elaboration, and refinement of hypotheses about the organization and its problems. It has been our experience that, as client and consultant work together, many further valuable data are fed into the study, since the client increasingly realizes the relevance of his own experience in the organization and recognizes the potential therapeutic benefits of frank communication. Quite significant reorientations tend to take place, during such work, in the views of individuals about themselves, their colleagues, and the organization, and in their relationships to the organization and each other.

As to the choice of people to whom to report, one would wish to report to all people who are likely to be involved in the problem and in change subsequent to the report. In the case of large organizations, of course, it is often impossible to work directly with all the people concerned and one may have to work with representatives. The experience behind this preference for direct reporting is connected not only with the belief that, in principle, people should have some share in decisions that affect them, but also with the practical point that this again facilitates working through resistance to the acceptance of data and their implications and of changes that may be based on them.

In working towards some resolution of the organization's problems, it would not be usual for the consultant to make specific recommendations about what changes should be initiated. Rather, the consultant would try to help the people concerned in the organization to evolve new solutions for themselves, based on their own experience and on the research findings and their implications, and accepting the restraints existing in the nature of the organization and of the people in it. In other words, the process involved is essentially one whereby the organization itself is enabled to find new and more constructive ways of dealing with its tasks and problems, on the basis of improved information and increased insights on the one hand, and the lessening of barriers to effective communication and of resistance to change on the other.

In such circumstances the solutions found are not likely to be 'ideal' in the blueprint sense. As in individual or group psychotherapy, the changes will go only as far as the client organization and the consultant can take them in the current circumstances. It is pointless to try to impose solutions that the organization could not operate or that its environment would not permit. Such an attempt would be likely only to increase resistance to change.

Finally, there is the question of the termination of the therapeutic relationship between the client organization and the consultant. It is, in our experience, important for the successful completion of the work that the relationship continue throughout the difficult phase of planning change and dealing with the disturbances inevitable in accomplishing it. It seems to us inappropriate that the consultant should behave as too many do, that is, write his prescription for social change and leave the organization alone to face the consequences of trying to implement the prescription. When the consultant *should* withdraw is much harder to define than when he should not. When he does is partly a matter of his socioclinical judgement as to when the organization is sufficiently stabilized to carry on without further help; partly it is a matter of meeting and dealing with the organization's own wishes. It is not uncommon for the relationship of client and consultant to go on intermittently for an indefinite period, to give support and help with problems as they arise. The consultant walks a tight-rope between withholding desirable help and colluding with over-dependency, which may arise in an organization just as in individual patients.

THE HOSPITAL STUDY
AS AN ILLUSTRATION OF THESE METHODS

The initiative for this study came from the hospital itself, the matron having been advised by a nursing colleague that the Tavistock Institute might be able to help her to deal more effectively with problems in the nurse training system, namely, in the allocation of student nurses to practical training and nursing duties. The study stemmed, therefore, from the practical needs of the hospital rather than from the consultant's wish to study hospitals, although in fact the Institute was very glad to have the opportunity to do research in a hospital.

There followed a series of exploratory discussions between the

matron, the deputy matron, the assistant matrons, and the principal tutor for the hospital and members of the senior staff of the
Tavistock Institute. This group decided provisionally to go ahead
with the study under the direction of the author. However, the
group felt that it would be desirable before making a final decision to consult other nurses who would be involved in the study.
Accordingly, meetings were held with other nursing staff and
with representatives of the student nurses. The aim of these meetings was to explain the purpose and methods of the proposed
study, to allow the nurses to express their views, doubts, and
questions, and to seek their support and collaboration in the study.
Such support being forthcoming, a final decision was made to go
ahead.

It would be idle to suppose that much more than formal support
was given at that stage. It would not, in fact, have been easy for
either staff or student nurses to challenge the tentative decision of
the senior staff to undertake the study. Such a challenge would not
have been in line with nursing tradition. On the other hand, the
meetings did allow the people concerned to get to know a little
about the study and the consultant, and gave them some feeling
that we were prepared to be influenced by the social field in which
we worked. This facilitated later, more comprehensive working
through of doubts and difficulties about the study.

The next task was to plan and to carry out the diagnostic survey.
We interviewed, either individually or in small groups, almost all
the qualified nurses in the hospital, some of them many times. We
interviewed individually and in small groups a 10 per cent sample
of the student nurses. We also interviewed a few of the senior
medical staff and the senior lay administrators. We carried out
observational studies of four contrasting wards. In addition, we
collected a good deal of statistical data relevant to the problem of
allocation of student nurses to practical training and nursing
duties.

As we became known and our guarantee of anonymity and
confidentiality became reasonably well trusted, we found that our
informants were prepared to talk very frankly and fully about their
experiences and we could begin to build a relatively comprehensive picture of the nursing situation in the hospital. As soon
as we felt fairly well informed about the situation, we initiated the
more 'therapeutic' activities. We began by reporting verbally to

the matron, but very soon, with her agreement, we broadened the basis of this reporting to a group consisting of the five senior nurses in the hospital. This group met at approximately fortnightly intervals over some months, each meeting lasting two to three hours. At first, the meetings consisted largely of verbal reporting by the consultant, but later they became much more a general pooling of experience and views by all the members of the group. Much valuable diagnostic material emerged from the contributions of the nurses from their long and rich experience in nursing.

These meetings were an exciting and moving therapeutic experience. The process in the group resembled the process in a therapeutic group, although its objective was social change and was not directly concerned with the individual members as such. A great deal of the work was concerned with working through resistance to the acceptance of the contributions made both by individual members and by the study, and with following up the implications of these contributions. The group worked on the material provided within itself; examined contributions; checked and rechecked their validity in the light of its combined experience; contradicted, elaborated, and refined them. Quite significant reorientation took place in the group and in individuals with regard to the problems we were tackling together, and in the relationships between the members of the group. In particular, the group developed a greater capacity for free interchange of views than is usual in a senior nursing group. The courage and sincerity of the group in tackling the difficult problems of change in a notably rigid profession were most impressive.

The group gradually crystallized out of its discussions several plans for change in the system of allocating student nurses to practical training and nursing duties and in surrounding areas of their work. The implementation of such plans obviously involved other nursing staff and students, and they now began to be involved also in the sociotherapeutic process. The suggested plans were put to their representatives and were explored by them and modified in certain ways before finally being put into operation.

The therapeutic process was not, of course, confined to formal situations in which the consultant took part. A vast amount of work was also done by nursing staff and students in other situations and then fed back into the formal planning meetings. This work was sometimes done in formal meetings or in the carrying

out of various preparatory tasks such as devising a plan for
student-nurse allocation. But a great deal of it was informal talking, done in off-duty periods and as the nurses went about their
ordinary duties. One of the notable things about this sort of study
is the extent to which it stimulates thinking and exploration in the
client organization itself.

There was a gradual reduction in frequency of contact between
the consultant and the nursing staff as the plans evolved and the
nurses themselves took over their implementation. The study
proper stopped when the plans were implemented and the new
situation around them seemed to have stabilized, although some
casual contact between the senior nursing staff and the consultant continued for some time afterwards.

I should like to mention in concluding this account of the study
a particular serious limitation from which it suffered. It did not
prove possible for a number of reasons effectively to involve in
the study the other two main social sub-systems in the hospital,
namely, medical and lay. This meant, in effect, that change in the
nursing system was limited to such changes as could be introduced
without requiring any major balancing adjustments in the other
sub-systems. It would not have been possible, for example, to
bring about any major change in ward organization without the
full cooperation of the medical staff because of its effect on the
medical sub-system.

CONCLUDING REMARKS

This paper has described one particular research approach out of
many possible approaches. My choice of this method of approach
is partly a matter of personal preference. I prefer to work in an
organization which has delineated a problem in its own functioning and has a real drive towards social change. In other words, I
personally prefer a clinical and therapeutic relationship with the
organization being studied. To achieve this, I am prepared to be
directed by the field as regards the organization and the problem
to be studied.

As a research method, this clinical approach has both advantages and disadvantages compared with other available research
methods. To comment only briefly on this point, our experience
has been that the therapeutic relationship with the client organization tends to facilitate access to significant data in their full com-

plexity and depth. This is connected with informants' motivation for communication, which stems to a considerable extent from the drive towards the resolution of problems and social change. Such motivation creates a very different situation from that in which the motivation stems from the research worker's need to do research. It has been our experience that, as the relevant connections are made between communication and problem-solving, the clinical approach encourages frankness in the informants and helps them to disclose intimate and painful facts in very much the same way as happens in individual or group psychotherapy. The informants' perspectives are also broadened and they begin to see the relevance of a wide range of experiences to the problem being tackled, and to be able to communicate on a broad front and in depth. These developments become particularly evident in the therapeutic phases of the study, which often provide the most significant research data.

A difficulty of the clinical approach lies in the very depth and complexity of the data it provides, factors that may make the analysis and interpretation of the data a hazardous task compared with the analysis and interpretation of data from more structured research approaches. Understanding depends greatly on what the consultant can himself make of the data, and is therefore subject to the risk of his misunderstanding because of subjective factors in himself. Checks can be provided, however, to minimize this risk, e.g. in the form of constant interchange between members of the consultant team or 'supervision' from other experienced colleagues outside the study, and of constant checking and rechecking in the field. The understanding of the data is also a stressful task for the consultant, since it depends so much on his internalizing the data and on his emotional, as well as his intellectual, sifting processes. The data have to be 'felt' inside oneself; that is, one has to take in and experience the stress in the organization, much as one does in individual and group psychotherapy. This is very different from a situation which has all the external supports of such devices as structured questionnaires and sophisticated statistical techniques for analysing data.

A disadvantage of the method lies also in the limitation it imposes on the choice of research problems. This obviously makes it necessary to devise and use other methods of approach to problems where, from the social point of view, research patently

needs to be done but the chances that anyone will bring the matter
to a research worker are not great. Many of the more diffuse problems of our society – e.g. geriatric problems or road accidents –
do not lend themselves to such an approach, since the people who
need help are not organized to seek it.

On the other hand, the disadvantages are to some extent balanced by the valuable and sometimes unexpected by-products that
emerge from such studies. The access so gained to an organization
has on a number of occasions enabled the consultant to increase
the general understanding and theoretical formulations about the
functioning of social systems. In the hospital study we were
fortunate in working in an organization, the nature of whose task,
caring for the sick, stimulated a great deal of anxiety and stress in
the members of the organization. The data collected around this
situation enabled us further to develop theoretical formulations
put forward by other authors in relation to one particular aspect
of the functioning of social systems, namely, their use by their
members as socially structured systems of defence against anxiety.
These socially structured defence systems not only affect the
emotional satisfactions and difficulties of the members of the
organization, but can be shown to affect also the efficiency and
viability of the organization as such. An understanding of the
anxieties and the social defence systems adds an important
dimension to the total understanding of social organizations and
to diagnostic and therapeutic work within them.

REFERENCES

BION, W. R. (1961). *Experiences in groups, and other papers*. London:
    Tavistock Publications; New York: Basic Books.
JAQUES, E. (1953). On the dynamics of social structure. *Hum.
    Relat.* **6**, 3–24.
MENZIES, I. E. P. (1960a). A case-study in the functioning of
    social systems as a defence against anxiety: a report on a study
    of the nursing service of a general hospital. *Hum. Relat.* **13**,
    95–121.
—— (1960b). Nurses under stress. *Internat. nursing Rev.* **7**, No. 6,
    9–16. Also published in *Nursing Times* (1961) **57**, 141–2,
    173–4, 206–7.

—— (1965). Some mutual interactions between organizations and their members. (Paper read at the 6th International Congress of Psychotherapy, London, 1964.) *Psychother. Psychosom.* **13**, 194–200.

TRIST, E. L. & BAMFORTH, K. W. (1951). Some social and psychological consequences of the longwall method of coalgetting. *Hum. Relat.* **4**, 3–38.

Part III: Theoretical Approaches

7 Sociology and Psychiatry

NORBERT ELIAS

To clarify the relationship between psychiatry and sociology may, at first glance, appear an easy task. But the impression is deceptive. Both are concerned with the study of human beings; but we have at present no clear theoretical model showing how the various sciences of men fit into each other. In fact, one of the reasons for the difficulties one encounters if one attempts to clarify interdisciplinary relationships is the total inadequacy for such a task of the philosophical theories of science which still largely dominate thinking in this field. They still proceed as if classical physics is the eternal model to which all other scientific studies should look for guidance. The English word 'science' itself has a ring about it which suggests that not much has happened in the field of science since the seventeenth or eighteenth century. It is only very slowly that the meaning of the word science begins to adjust itself to the various types of scientific specialism that have developed since then and are multiplying at an increasing rate. It is now possible to speak – perhaps still a little shamefacedly – of human sciences or of social sciences. But even in my own field hardly any investigation exists into the conditions and the reasons for increasing scientific specialization, or into its consequences. For some time I have taken an interest in this theme, in the practical and theoretical problems of increasing scientific specialization, and particularly in the relations between different scientific specialisms.

Psychiatry and sociology are two of the many specialisms concerned with the study of men. As scientific disciplines go, both are fairly young. But already new specialisms, such as social psychiatry and group psychotherapy, begin to sprout in the no-man's land between them, reinforcing the need for closer cooperation. However, despite the ease with which the word 'interdisciplinary' rolls off our tongues, in practice the establishment

of closer cooperation, or simply of better communication, between different professional groups of scientific specialists encounters some basic difficulties which are easily overlooked. A
good deal of preparatory reflection is needed if the efforts required
are to be fruitful. To some extent, my paper will be concerned
with this task.

I thought it might be best to set out first some of these difficulties. They themselves are examples of the kind of problem
with which sociologists are concerned. For in order to explain
these difficulties, one has to investigate the relations between the
professional groups to which the individuals concerned belong,
that is, between psychiatrists and sociologists. One cannot explain
such difficulties in terms of distinguishing personal characteristics
of these individuals. Practitioners in both fields usually share with
their fellow practitioners certain basic modes of thinking and
certain basic attitudes, particularly in relation to those who, from
their point of view, are outsiders or 'lay people'. They identify
themselves with their profession. Through training, work, and
social contacts with fellow practitioners, they usually acquire
common professional characteristics as an integral part of their
individual personality. Their professional group is one of the
character-forming reference groups of which they say 'we'. And
for an adult in societies such as ours, this we-experience, the
identification with an occupational specialism, forms – for those
who have received a specialized training – as integral an aspect of
their self as the aspects to which they refer as 'I'.

As a result, the relationship between the professional groups
in the macrocosm of society projects itself into the relationship
between their individual practitioners if they meet professionally –
for example, in order to discuss interdisciplinary problems. If one
of two professional groups claims a higher standing than the
other, its individual representatives in meeting those of the other
will probably treat them with courtesy, as befits civilized human
beings, but also with a measure of reserve and perhaps con-
descension. If the two professional groups in society at large are
engaged, as often happens, in a status struggle, the tension is
likely to make itself felt in the encounters of their individual
representatives. Representatives of different scientific disciplines
are usually very conscious of status differences which exist between
their professions. And, as in the case of status differences between

different nations, the status of a particular scientific discipline among other scientific disciplines is closely connected with differences in the amount of power that their professional representatives as a collective body can wield within the various scientific and academic institutions and in society at large. Power differentials between different scientific disciplines and their professional representatives are substantial. Moreover, as in other occupational sectors of industrial societies, considerable mobility exists in the standing of scientific disciplines. New specialisms rise, older ones decline in standing and in power. Perhaps in no other type of society have the incidence of occupational specialization and the mobility, the upward and downward movement of the social standing of occupations, been so great as they are in ours, and, with them, the general status insecurity of the representatives of these occupations. As far as one can see, only members of old and wealthy aristocratic houses appear reasonably immune, and – perhaps – groups of unskilled labourers, and others concerned more with their daily bread and with amenities than with problems of status. Otherwise status anxieties and status insecurities are among the most ubiquitous characteristics of societies with a rapid proliferation of new, and a corresponding threat to the standing of old, specialisms.

This is certainly the case with newly emerging branches of scientific specialisms. Their professional representatives have almost invariably to struggle for recognition, for equality of standing, for a share in the professional rewards of status, finance, and prestige, with older and longer-established scientific and academic groups. The pioneers responsible for the development and advance in Britain of relatively new branches of medicine such as social psychiatry and group psychotherapy are probably not unfamiliar with such problems, and they are to be congratulated on their success in establishing a special Section of the greatly respected Royal Medico-Psychological Association for their young disciplines.

But some readers may well remember the longer struggle for recognition, equality of status, and a share in institutional power and opportunities, that took place between psychiatrists as a professional group and representatives of the older, already firmly established branches of medicine. The members of my own profession of sociology have been for some time engaged in a similar struggle with older academic specialisms; it has been a particularly difficult and long-drawn-out struggle in Britain – more difficult, in fact, than in any other country at a comparable stage of development. And although it has resulted in a rather sudden institutional expansion, the typical tensions surrounding a rising discipline continue.

Status differentials and the associated status tensions and status anxieties contribute a great deal to the problems that can be observed in all cases where a growing discipline calls, as the work of social psychiatry does, for collaboration between different disciplines that previously had few, if any, institutional contacts. There are many precedents for specialisms that start on their way as a kind of hybrid in the previously unexplored no-man's land between two already established specialisms: biochemistry, now clearly recognized as a specialism in its own right, is an example. The problems arising from such a fusion of different scientific specialisms are far-reaching. As a subject of study they themselves belong to a special branch of sociology – the sociology of knowledge – and may give an idea of its task.

Each of the previously independent professional groups – let us say psychiatrists and sociologists – whose collaboration is required in a newly rising specialized field, such as group psychotherapy or social psychiatry, has a theoretical framework of its own. Each has its own research and teaching methods, its own institutional traditions, and its own technical language. This last is all the more likely to cause difficulties of communication between the two groups, since the technical language of each group of specialists serves as a symbol of their professional status and skill in relation to outsiders, in addition to serving as a vehicle of precise communication within the group.

Moreover, in many cases scientific specialisms have – in connection with their special theoretical frame of reference – an exclusive mode of explaining phenomena. And if both are concerned, as they are in this case, with the study of human beings, the explanations for which they look, and which they may at first put forward as hypothetical solutions for problems of common interest, are liable to clash. One might say – for example's sake – that psychiatrists would try to explain in terms of sibling rivalries what sociologists would try to explain in terms of status rivalries, or in terms of self-destructive personality structures what sociologists would try to explain in terms of social anomie – and both may be partly right.

The difficulty is that, as in other similar cases, each group of scientific specialists regards its own type of explanation as exhaustive and exclusive. Hence a curious situation arises if members of two of these groups try to communicate. Faced with related problems, each offers its own type of explanation. In a sense the two groups become involved in a competitive struggle, each attempting to reduce the other's explanation to its own as the more fundamental type. They may be too civil to bring these differences into the open, but, whether they say it or not, each of the two sides thus brought face to face in an interdisciplinary exchange or in an attempt to collaborate may easily experience the other as amateurish or – less consciously – as a threat to its own professional skill. Each may feel that the other group threatens its own professional and theoretical autonomy.

This is a crucial point. In most cases the status of a scientific profession is closely bound up with its ability to develop types of concepts, of models, of explanations – in short, a theoretical framework of its own. The autonomy of the theoretical framework serves as legitimization of that of the scientific profession itself. It is the guarantor – or perhaps one should say the fortress wall – that secures the relative independence of one group of scientific specialists in relation to others.

In fact, recognition of the fruitfulness of the relatively autonomous theoretical models of a scientific specialism plays no small part in the social recognition of its status among academic disciplines. Hence one can observe a strong tendency in almost all scientific specialisms, and most of all in those that are relatively new and uncertain of their own standing, to overemphasize the degree of their theoretical autonomy and to disguise or to neglect their theoretical and practical interdependence with other specialisms. One could point to a number of instances in which claims to an autonomous theoretical framework have been put forward by an academic specialism on slender grounds as part of its quest for recognition as an independent academic discipline with its own institutional trappings; and to others in which a high degree of status insecurity on the part of the members of an academic discipline is closely associated with insecurities and disputes about its theoretical foundations.

I am using the problem with which we are most immediately concerned, that of the relationship of psychiatry and sociology, as an object lesson in the sociologists' approach to such problems. I have tried to give the briefest outline of a chapter in a sociology of sciences which itself forms part of a special branch of sociology, the sociology of knowledge. It can serve as a further illustration of the differences between, but also of the possible interdependence of, the psychiatrists' and the sociologists' approaches to cognate problems. Let us consider the imaginary case of acute anxiety states in a member of an academic profession with built-in status insecurities and recurrent status struggles with representatives of neighbouring academic disciplines. There may well be a certain affinity between the personality structure and the social structure of the profession. Whichever it is, a psychiatrist's diagnosis and, perhaps even more, his therapeutic prescription would be incomplete if they were not informed by a clear sociological diagnosis of these and other aspects of a person's occupation. One encounters here a still largely unexplored problem area of social psychiatry.

It may need fairly sustained exchanges of experiences and views between psychiatrists and sociologists over a period of time before effective techniques for the solution of interdependent problems can be worked out. Collaboration of this kind is made difficult, as I have mentioned before, by the tendency of each side to regard its own type of explanation as exclusive and all-embracing. Interdisciplinary discussions between representatives of disciplines with competing models of explanation rest on an unsafe basis. They can be effectively blocked as long as problems such as these are not made explicit and are not openly discussed. This, as you can see, is what I am trying to do.

All the various difficulties of communication between psychiatrists and sociologists, as between representatives of other human sciences, converge on a central difficulty. The specialists who are devoted to the scientific exploration of the human universe tend to build up from the limited segment of human beings under their care a unitary model of man on an all too narrow factual base. The best known of these parochial specialists' models of men is the *Homo economicus*. But one can observe in other social sciences equally parochial models of men. Thus psychiatrists make certain common assumptions about men in general, which reflect their circumscribed professional experiences. These permeate their procedures, their concepts, their whole mode of thinking about men. The same can be said of psychologists or of sociologists. One could speak of a *Homo psychiatricus*, a *Homo psychoanalyticus*, or a *Homo sociologicus*.

All of these groups are inclined to see their own province of the human universe as the most basic and the most central. As a result, those aspects with which they are professionally concerned stand out sharply and highly structured in the foreground of their image of men; other aspects that lie beyond their own field of studies and outside their own control are usually perceived as part of an unstructured background.

In the psychiatrist's perception, as I see it, the single individual – the single patient – stands out sharply in the foreground. All other people connected with him are perceived as a more or less unstructured background. The terms habitually used underline and reinforce this structure of the psychiatrist's perception and the picture of man that goes with it. It is not unusual to speak of a patient's 'social background'; one may speak of a child's 'bad background' if one means his family; or, worse still, one may speak of family, neighbourhood, community, and other similar social configurations as a person's 'environment'. In the eyes of many sociologists, by contrast, all these configurations are highly structured. One can study the structure of neighbourhoods and communities, and the structure of the families that live there. I myself have once undertaken such a study (Elias & Scotson, 1965). Nor can I doubt that many psychiatrists are aware – if not with regard to neighbourhoods or occupations, at least with regard to families – that a person's relations with others are open to a fairly rigorous analysis. In point of fact, they often make attempts to determine the configuration of, say, husband, wife, elder son, and younger daughter in a particular case. But their training does not equip them too well for a systematic exploration of family structures. It expresses the implied evaluation of their concept of man that, by comparison with the individual with whom they are concerned, the network of relationships of which the individual forms part, all the social structures to which he belongs, come under the heading 'environmental factors'. The terminology itself implies the existence of a wall between the highly structured person in the foreground and the seemingly unstructured network of relations and communications in the background.

In discussions between psychiatrists and sociologists that is one of the sources of misunderstandings. Whereas sociologists, speaking of families or of groups and societies in general, may refer to what they perceive as configurations of people with structures, and often also with dynamics, of their own, psychiatrists may take up the sociologists' argument in terms of highly structured individuals with relatively unstructured 'backgrounds', without awareness of the difference. One can see at once the importance, for any collaborative effort in fields such as social psychiatry and group psychotherapy, of this confrontation between differences in the basic concepts, and of the evaluation of data that follow from them.

As a theoretical model, the *Homo psychiatricus* is based on the assumption of a fairly radical division between what goes on 'inside' and what goes on 'outside' the individual human being. The vocabulary of a psychiatric diagnosis, like that of a physical medical diagnosis, refers almost exclusively to the former; it refers to supposedly 'internal' processes of man, such as compulsion syndromes, object cathexis, perversion, and character disorders, which seem to run their course with almost complete autonomy in relation to the 'environment', to the network of relationships and communications of one human being with others.

The *Homo psychiatricus*, then, is a human being stripped of most attributes which one might call 'social', such as attributes connected with the standing of his family, with his educational attainments, his occupational training and work, or his national characteristics and identifications. The individual person is seen essentially as a closed system whose own internal processes have a high degree of independence in relation to what appear as 'external' or social factors. In general, the latter are evaluated as peripheral when a person is considered psychiatrically. They can be 'taken off', as it were, like a patient's clothes in a doctor's surgery.

The presentation of the psychiatrist's concept of man would be incomplete if one did not add that the *Homo psychiatricus* is in many respects a more sophisticated and refined version of the dominant concept of man of contemporary industrial societies as a *Homo clausus*. In these societies, terms such as 'group' or 'society' are very widely used as if they refer to something that lies outside of man, that surrounds or 'environs' the single individual.

The image evoked by these conventions of speaking and thinking is that of a high wall surrounding the single individual, from which mysterious little dwarfs – the 'environmental influences' – throw small rubber balls at the individual, which leave on him some imprints. That is the way in which terms like 'social factors' and others of this kind are commonly employed.

It is, as one can see, the perspective of a human being who experiences himself alone at the centre of things, while everything else lies outside, separated from him by an invisible wall, and who imputes as a matter of course the same experience to all other individuals. From this basic experience of oneself as a somewhat lonely and isolated person, as the centre of all others, one arrives at the general concept of 'the individual' in the singular as the centre of the human world. This individual-centred perspective of the human universe is in many ways the contemporary counterpart of the former geocentric perspective of the natural universe.

For many people today it is difficult to imagine that other forms of human self-awareness are at all possible. However, the perception of oneself and of others as single individuals, each of whom experiences himself as the centre of the human universe and all other people as something outside, is not very old. It is confined to a group of fairly advanced European and American societies during a limited period of their development, and even during that period, in all likelihood, mainly to the educated elites. The strong conviction it carries as something immediately intelligible in societies such as these is itself closely connected with the specific structure and development of these societies. There is no need in this context to go further. But it may be useful to say that one of the contributory factors is certainly the very firm hold that this experience, since it began to assert itself towards the end of the Middle Ages, has gained over the vocabulary of these societies. Today, the verbal carriers of this perspective are handed on from one generation to another as a common currency of discourse and, as such, are apt to reinforce other factors in our manner of living which help to cast our self-experience in that particular mould. Who would think of questioning the appropriateness of such phrases as 'the individual and his environment' or 'individual and society', which almost make it appear that one is speaking of two different objects?

However, it is not uninteresting to remember that the dusk of

the geocentric view of the natural universe coincided with the
dawn of the individual-centred view of man and the human
universe. Thus John Donne in his great poem 'The first anni-
versarie' (published 1611), in which he – at the beginning of one
of the greatest periods in the history of England and of Europe –
sadly contemplated the general decay of the world, and referred
to the rising individual-centredness of man as a symptom of that
decay. Almost in the same breath in which he alluded to the new
heliocentric philosophy, which, as he saw it, 'cast all in doubt' so
that no one any longer knew where earth and sun stood, and
'all coherence was gone', he complained that:

> *. . . every man alive thinkes he hath got*
> *To be a Phoenix, and that there can bee*
> *None of that kinde, of which he is, but hee.*

In retrospect, people sometimes appear to find it difficult to
understand why their ancestors clung so long to a geocentric
view and could not see its inadequacies, which seem today to be
obvious. One is hardly any longer aware what depth of disillusion-
ment followed the doubts cast by the rising natural sciences on
the cherished position of man's good earth as the centre of God's
universe. Nor does one often remember the courage of the great
scientific pioneers who felt that they could no longer conform to
the ruling views of their time and who fought – often at considerable personal risk – for their deviant ideas of nature against
the still solid phalanx of the established geocentric beliefs.

The comparison between the very strong conviction once
carried by the geocentric picture of the physical universe – which
at its core was also an anthropocentric picture – and the equally
strong conviction carried today, particularly in the more developed
societies, by an individual-centred picture of the human universe,
may make it easier to see the latter in perspective.

Unless one is able to stand back and to distance oneself from
the individual-centred form of self-awareness, it is difficult to
understand the difference between the psychiatrists' and the
sociologists' concepts of man. I could not blame anyone for
thinking that a sociologist would wish to replace the individual-
centred by a society-centred concept of man. However, as they
are used today, 'individual' and 'society' are concepts of the same
kind. If one is able to dissociate oneself from the terminological

convention of one's own time, one can see that both terms in their present form draw a veil over our eyes; they agree very little with what we actually observe if we study human beings with a measure of detachment. They make it appear that there are individuals outside society and a society outside individuals; that these two entities, the 'individual without society' and the 'society without individuals', stand in the same relation to each other as do two different physical objects – we say 'individual and society interact' as if they were two billiard balls – and that they are in some sense even antithetical towards each other. As symbols of specific emotional experiences, such as the feeling of personal frustration through social norms, or of political ideals, such as capitalism and socialism, these two terms may well assume the meaning of opposites. But the sociologist's task, as I see it, is that of working out a concept of men which is influenced neither by political slogans of the age nor by the type of self-experience that makes it appear that oneself is in some way alone, separated from all others 'outside' by an almost impenetrable wall. The capacity to detach oneself from that type of experience and from the modes of thinking based on it is the crucial condition for any break with petrified traditions of thinking and acting. But its realization in depth is not easy. It demands a far-reaching reorganization of one's perception and different concepts to express it.

If one has gained sufficient distance one can see that all individual human beings form with each other specific configurations: families, towns, churches, business enterprises, battles, football games, nations, therapeutic groups, and innumerable others – all in a slow or rapid state of flux and all connected with others. But it is not enough to perceive other people forming configurations of various types. The decisive step is to perceive also oneself as a part of such configurations, as one among others, as an interdependent individual.

Today it is still rather difficult to stand back far enough to perceive individuals, and among them oneself, forming configurations with each other which have regularities, structures, and dynamics of their own, so that one can see at the same time the personality structures and dynamics of the individuals who form these configurations and those of the configurations themselves as inseparable, but distinct, levels of events.

One of the main reasons for the difficulty is the sharp division habitually made today between what goes on 'inside' and what goes on 'outside' men – between 'endogenous' and 'exogenous' processes. As expression of a specific type of self-experience, which is common in the more developed societies of our time, the sharp division between what goes on 'within' a person and what goes on 'without' is justified. As a factual statement about human beings, it is not. If one is able to distance oneself sufficiently from this self-experience, its fantasy character becomes apparent. The notion of an invisible wall separating one individual from another, and the whole family of concepts based on the idea that the 'essential' self of one individual is hidden away 'within' from that of all others, are by no means shared by men of all human societies; they develop in and through specific types of relationship between individuals, characteristic of the conditions of life in specific societies. Small children have no 'walls' of this kind, or, to be more precise, no self-experience of such walls. Nor do they grow as part of men's nature automatically.

Comparisons between different societies indicate that the feeling of aloneness, of isolation, of the ultimate separation and independence of oneself in relation to other individuals, which finds expression in the concept of the individual that prevails today – of the individual human being as a closed system with his essentials hidden away from others 'inside' – is lacking in many other, particularly in simpler, societies where privatization of bodily functions and of feeling is neither possible nor socially required to the same extent as in ours. There is good reason to think that the feeling of oneself as a closed system, with all its conceptual representations, is symptomatic of the strength, the evenness, and the all-roundness of the social restraints that are built into the emerging individual in societies such as ours through specific types of social pressure as much as through deliberate family training. It is, one might say, an expression of a particular conscience formation bred in particular societies.[1]

What kind of image of man comes into sight if one is able to stand back far enough to perceive individuals and among them oneself forming configurations with each other which have regularities, structures, and dynamics of their own, so that one can see at the same time the dynamics and structures of the individuals and those of the configurations they form as inseparable, but distinct?

Throughout life every human being is linked to others by numerous ties. If these links wither, he as a person becomes impoverished and withers too. The only human beings to whom the concept of man as a basically closed system might apply are some types of severely psychotic people. In their case the psychiatrists' efforts are directed towards opening, as far as possible, the blocked channels of communication with others. Psychotherapy in all its various forms is a social process involving two or more people. It aims at restoring, at redirecting or developing, valencies of feeling and affective acting towards others so that communication through speech and other forms of behaviour can flow more realistically or, as we say, more normally. Thus the theoretical tradition of psychotherapy largely based on the closed-system model of man stands askance to the practice of psychotherapy which is aimed at reorganizing, rechannelling, and reopening, if blocked, libidinal, affective, and intellectual valencies directed from one person towards others.

It requires a considerable effort to build up an adequate and realistic model of men as open systems, a bridge between the psychiatrists' and the psychologists' traditional problem area and that of sociologists. Perhaps one can best indicate the direction of the changes in thinking about men that become necessary if the closed-system model of the individual and the inside/outside dichotomy are given up, by an example which is within the range of the experience of most people: the death of a loved person. Would one regard this as something that happens outside the person concerned as distinct from that which happens inside? Would one classify it as environmental?

This is the way in which this type of event has been classified by J. L. Halliday (1948) in *Psychosocial medicine*.[2] He distinguishes 'the field of the person' from 'the field of environment' and lists among the examples of environmental psychological causes of illnesses, together with 'failure of promotion', 'death of a loved person'. And in his view as in that of others the distinction between 'person' and 'environment' as two separate and different 'fields' of events goes hand in hand with a specific concept of causation. The environment is treated as one agent, the person as another. The former acts upon the latter more or less in the same way in which a moving billiard ball acts upon another at rest which it encounters at a given time on a billiard table. 'Person' and 'the event in the environment' are treated as if they were two different objects on the same level which are up to a certain time unconnected; one of them as a cause, it seems, by connecting with the other at a given moment in time, produces a specific effect – the illness.

One can easily see how little this traditional scheme of explanation corresponds to what one actually observes in this situation. The effect of which the death of the loved person is the 'cause' can hardly be described in terms of an 'encounter' between a person and something 'environmental' – something that comes, like a bacillus or a falling brick, from 'outside' the person. Nor can this death of another person be adequately described as a 'social' event, distinct from 'psychological' or 'individual' events, or as an 'exogenous' in contrast to an 'endogenous' cause of illness. The phenomenon of a love attachment defies conceptualization in terms of these conventional dichotomies. All attempts at coming to grips with this type of connection between persons according to the classical models of physical causality – in terms of the types of connection learned from observation of inanimate bodies – are insufficient. This does not mean that one has to resign oneself to metaphysical explanations. It is not beyond the intellectual resources of man to develop clear theoretical models and concepts that fit the nexus of events to be observed in this case more closely than those we have.

Love relationships – like other human relationships – can be seen, at the same time, in two ways: with the eyes of non-participants, who can speak and think of the people concerned as THEY, and with the eyes of the participants who, speaking of their relationships, can say WE. The traditional concepts that are used to express the distinction and the relationship between these two perspectives hardly bear closer examination. One may perhaps classify the THEY-perspective as 'objective', the I- or WE-perspective as 'subjective', but then one is burdened with the spectre of the old epistemological mythology which postulates an eternal gulf between the closed system of the individual 'subject' and the world of 'objects' outside. If anything, a love relationship between two people is subjective and objective at the same time. It is better to abandon old linguistic traditions burdened with a philosophical heritage that is beginning to become obsolete.

To speak of dimensions, levels, perspectives, in accordance with the various positions indicated by the series of personal pronouns, may be found more appropriate. In terms of the THEY-perspective, a love relationship is a specific configuration of people. As such it has its specific dynamics, which are determined as much by the structure of society at large as by that of the two constituents of that society most immediately concerned. But one cannot quite understand configurations of people from the THEY-perspective without taking into account that these people themselves also experience these configurations from a different, from the I- or WE-, perspective. Of these configurations, love relations, friendships, enmities, and other affective relationships have in this context a special significance. As a problem area they constitute, whatever we make of it, a no-man's land or a link between psychiatry and sociology.

Perhaps one can best conceptualize this aspect of men by saying that each individual has open valencies ready to connect with those of other individuals according to a schema whose groundwork has been laid by his early childhood experiences in the family, which have been further elaborated by his emotional experiences as a constituent of other configurations. Gradually, a more firmly set configuration of valencies directed towards others will develop. Some may be firmly bound to those of another person in a lasting reciprocal affective relationship, while others may remain open as strivings, as scanning valencies, bound only by transient link-ups or bound to relatively impersonal objectives such as occupational activities, hobbies, and causes, or perhaps to specific fantasy figures.

Some current theories give the impression that only one valency is, as it were, beamed from one individual towards another, the sexual valency. But if perception is not dimmed by any theoretical dogmatism, this is hardly what one observes. The types of an individual's relationships with others involving affective valencies, a striving for the dovetailing with those of other persons, are much more numerous and varied. However mutually satisfactory a long-lasting monogamous marriage relationship may be as a sexual partnership, it demands for its permanent maintenance much more than that. It is doubtful whether a marriage partnership catering successfully for the sex needs of husband and wife alone could satisfactorily absorb all the valencies of the two partners, all their needs for affective relationships and stimulation through contact with human beings; whether, in short, all the varied valencies of an individual could be satisfactorily concentrated in the relationship with *one* other person. There is a good deal of evidence to suggest that even a permanent one man/one woman relationship can be satisfactorily maintained only if one partner or both have non-sexual relationships, friendships, rivalries, pet enmities, professional or leisure-time contacts, which correspond at least in part and in varying degrees to emotional strivings towards other people as well. Whether one considers the child's imperative striving for stimulation through physical contact and communication with other human beings or the hardly less imperative need for affectionate human company, or whether one considers the mature adult's needs for a sexual partner as well as for non-sexual friendships or enmities, as the case may be, or perhaps for children, the valencies directed from one human being towards others are numerous and varied. The concept of a personal configuration of valencies characteristic of each individual, of which sexual valencies are one core type, corresponds to observations of this kind. Quite apart from its diagnostic function, it points to a basic problem of common interest to psychiatrists and to sociologists – to the problem of the connection between the personal configuration of valencies that the individual members of a society hold out towards each other and the configurations that that society, by virtue of its overall structure, requires individuals to form with each other.

A love relationship[3] constitutes one of the ways in which two individuals' valencies connect and dovetail into each other. As an example, it demonstrates most graphically the ineptitude of the model of man as a closed system, and of all its derivatives; it points in a simple way to the incongruousness of a conceptualization that likens man to a strong-box with an 'inside' hermetically sealed off from what is 'outside'. It is not more than a factual statement that is capable of empirical verification to say that human beings have a variety of strivings directed towards dovetailing with those of other human beings and thus binding them to each other affectively through love or hatred, positive or negative feeling, or both. One can hardly think of any more striking illustration of man's almost permanent readiness for attachment to others, of the ever-present character of free valencies, than the phenomenon that has come to be known in psychiatry as 'transference'.

Whether or not the psychoanalytic explanation of the special form of a transference relationship in terms of an individual's childhood relationship with his parents is correct – there is certainly a large body of evidence in its favour – the phenomenon as such is significant for our general concept of men. The astonishing ease with which a transference relationship, an affective attachment, positive or negative as the case may be, can be established in relation to a doctor, a political leader, or a religious preacher, or to members of a therapeutic group and in many other situations, even in the case of people whose sexually toned valencies are securely anchored in marriage, appears to indicate large reserves of free or unattached valencies in many individuals, which may or may not be highly specialized.

There is much room for research, not only into the specific form, but into the general nature of the valencies. One does not know, for example, whether the personal readiness for affective attachments, the reserves of free valencies specialized or unspecialized, are equally large in all individuals, in women and in men, in different age groups, in different societies; or whether the reserves of unspecialized valencies remain the same; or whether the more specialized valencies, sexual or non-sexual, connect in a personally satisfying manner with the objectives for which they are specialized. Nor does one know much about the long-term development of an individual's configuration of valencies in its connection with the sequence of configurations which he socially forms with others from the simple, narrow, and relatively undifferentiated family configurations of early childhood, to the wider and more differentiated configurations of adolescence and adulthood, and again to the shrinking configurations of old age. Thus a configurational approach, by extending attention to the whole profile of a person's valencies throughout his development, with its recurrent as well as its changing patterns of affective attachment and conflict, provides a theoretical scheme for the formulation and study of problems concerning the connections between the individual and the group level of human beings.

One can now see more clearly why the closed-system approach, and the conceptual dichotomy person/environment associated with this approach, are inadequate if one is confronted with problems such as that of the death of a loved person. If this death is followed by the illness of the person who loves, the connection is different from that to which one applies the term 'cause' in the case of a moving billiard ball 'causing', through its impact upon another at rest, a specific change in the latter; the connection is different, too, from that which applies in the case of an infecting agent brought in from 'outside' a person as a 'cause' of that person's illness. The death of a loved person 'causes' illness only because it is a *loved* person who has died. It causes illness because it changes the pre-existing configuration formed by two persons, of whom at least one was deeply dependent on the other.

The example is symptomatic of the inadequacy of many of our traditional tools of thinking for the exploration of human phenomena. One is apt to treat these instruments, deeply embedded in the customary language, as sacrosanct. One allows them to dictate the manner in which one perceives and experiences events without deliberately examining their fitness for the task at hand. Many basic instruments of thinking, concepts, categories, theoretical models, are handed on almost unchanged from generation to generation. The result is a growing discrepancy between the socially available knowledge of details, particularly in many human sciences, and the concepts, the categories, and the models used to indicate their connections with each other.

The death of a loved person, and its connection with changes in the person who loved, is a case in point.

This is the situation. An individual's love quest, his affective striving, one of his open valencies, had homed on another person. And now this person is dead. Like a limb amputated, an integral element of his self has been wrenched off. Not only this single configuration, the relationship between the lover and the loved person, has changed. The whole network of relationships, the overall configuration formed by him with other individuals, is likely to change too. It is likely to change on both the 'social' and the 'individual' level. But if one uses these two concepts here, one uses them no longer in the usual sense. The two levels can be distinguished, but cannot be separated or treated as necessarily antagonistic. They are permanently interdependent.

On the social level, the survivor's position in relation to others may change because he moves house. He may be richer or poorer than before. As soon as one begins to examine in greater detail the changes in the network of human relationships of which the survivor forms part, however, one will find the distinction 'social' and 'individual' too crude. Both the configuration he actually forms with other persons and the configuration of valencies characteristic of him as a person, with its peculiar profile and its specific balances and tensions, may change. But they will change not as two separate fields of events that interact, but as two levels of one and the same field.

An outside observer, a sociologist or anthropologist, may select for attention the changes in the whole configuration formed by the person who loved with others, perhaps in relation to the customs, traditions, and laws of his society, or to his class, his status group, and the special circumstances of his kinship group; he may view the whole change primarily with the eyes of someone perceiving the individual constituents of the changing configuration, including the bereaved person himself, as THEY. Another observer, a psychiatrist or psychologist, may try to explore primarily the individual experience of the person who loved; he may see the changes in the configuration with the eyes of someone who himself experiences them as an involved participant, who looks at them from the I-perspective while at the same time perceiving this person as HE.[4] But however much a division of labour may help, in actual fact the changes that occur in the grouping of people following the death of a person to whom at least one of them was deeply attached can be understood only if one takes account of the THEY- and HE-aspect as well as of the WE- and I-aspect of the change. According to the semantic traditions one might have to speak in this case of the 'objective' and the 'subjective' aspects or perhaps of the 'social' and the 'personal' aspects. But all these more familiar terms, as one can see, give the impression of a duality and an opposition between separate entities, such as 'object' and 'subject' or 'society' and 'person'.

In many ways they are a liability rather than a help if one tries to clarify the relationship between those aspects of a change in the grouping of people with which sociologists are concerned and those with which psychiatrists are concerned. Perhaps one may find the personal pronouns, references to the THEY- and WE-aspect and to the HE- and I-aspect, more useful. At least they express clearly that people considered in the plural as groups or configurations and people considered in the singular are the same people; and although the structures and regularities that come in sight if one explores men in the plural and man in the singular are of a different type, the two aspects are interdependent even if they are in tension and lead to conflicts – which can happen, but is not always the case.

They are certainly inseparable. It is hard to believe that one can understand the change brought about by a death in the configuration of the people concerned if one confines one's attention to what are usually called social factors, such as changes in the family grouping or the household arrangements, inheritance problems, or changes in fortune and status – in short, to specific sections of the THEY-aspect – without any consideration for the I-aspect, for the way in which the individuals concerned, and above all someone deeply attached to the dead person, experience the change.

It is equally difficult to believe that one can understand the changes in the behaviour and experience of an individual who has suffered the loss of a loved person if one pays attention only to what one often calls his 'inner' processes, to what he himself experiences, to the experiential, the I-perspective; or if one, as is often the case, focuses attention on his feelings towards, on his relationship with, the loved person alone. If the loved person was his wife or his mother, his relationships with other relatives or with friends and acquaintances, private as well as professional, may be affected. The relationship with another person, formerly marginal in the configuration of his attachments, may assume a warmth it never had before. Again, he may now become estranged from another who played a special role in his relationship with the dead person, perhaps as a catalyst. For yet another person to whom he was attached through valencies with a predominantly negative charge – jealousy, hostility, rivalry, or whatever their specific colour – he may now begin to feel more positively. One can focus now on the change in what one may call for want of a better word the 'objective' aspect of the configuration, now on the change in its 'subjective' aspect – on its third-person and its first-person aspects; in actual fact the two aspects are interdependent and inseparable.

As a rule, sociologists do not appear to pay sufficient attention to those types of social bond that provide the closest contacts with the psychiatrist's field of work, namely to affective valencies directed from one person to another, to the elementary readiness of human beings to attach themselves to each other. Without this, no communication between human beings is possible, and an elementary condition of social as well as of individual life is missing. Not hostility and conflict, but the withdrawal of affects, the incapacity to send out valencies and to form attachments, leads to a total breakdown of social relations.

Psychiatrists are of course familiar with the facts to which I have just referred. But they do not conceptualize them in the way I have done. Their understandable preoccupation with the single patient, whom they rarely, if ever, encounter in his normal social setting, their training according to a medical tradition which concentrates attention on a single body and a number of other factors, makes them inclined to perceive what they see as symptoms or mechanisms of a single organism even if it is very obviously directed from one organism to another. They stop thinking and questioning, perhaps even feeling any interest, if the track of observations leads beyond the professionally prescribed field.

It may have been noticed that my conception of valencies bears some kinship to the Freudian term 'libido'. In fact I could have spoken of libidinal valencies instead of using the more general term affective valencies. But in his theoretical studies Freud was not very interested in the fact that libido, as he described it, was in many of its aspects directed from one human being to another. Nothing is more characteristic of the specific slant of Freud's conceptualizations than the fact that his quest for understanding human beings came to a halt when he approached in his explorations those aspects of human beings that he called 'reality'. This was his code name for what sociologists would call 'social' – for societies, for groups, for the configurations that individuals form with each other.

Freud was probably not quite aware that what he called reality had its own structure. It is true that by training and inclination he was not well equipped to explore these structures. Nor was it his task. His explorations within his professional limits were fruitful enough. However, as a result of these limitations, many of Freud's theoretical concepts suggest the existence of a wall between the 'internal' fantasies which he explored and the 'external' reality which he did not explore. His concepts, and in fact many other psychiatric concepts, are slanted in accordance with the

implicit belief in this non-existent wall. It is one of the manifestations of the belief in man as a closed system and has until now
greatly influenced the theory of psychotherapy. To some extent,
it has acted as a barrier to the development of those forms of
psychotherapy that allow men, within certain limits, to come face
to face with their own problems in a setting more closely akin to
that of reality, in a setting where they actually form configurations
with others and where their personal configuration of valencies
operates, not only in a two-polar doctor/patient configuration,
but as in 'real' life in a multipolar configuration: I am speaking of
group psychotherapy. In that setting the difference between
fantasy conduct and realistic conduct shows itself most strikingly
precisely because one can experience how the two incessantly
flow into each other, how interdependent they are. Here the conceptual wall between fantasy and reality, between what seems to
be inside and what outside a person, and between person and
person generally, reveals itself as an intellectual artefact. The
term 'configuration of valencies' is an example of the type of
concept that will be needed if this artefact is to be removed.

It is precisely in a group setting that one can directly observe
this interdependency between the changing fortunes of valencies
that are directed from person to person and of others that people
keep consciously or unconsciously to themselves – or, in more
traditional language, how fantasies change when reality changes
and reality changes when fantasies change. Moreover, it seems to
me, the concept of valencies agrees better than the term libido in
its present form with the fact that normally men's emotional bonds
have a group character; they have a variety of forms, from maternal and paternal affection to the various sexual and affectionate
bonds between men and women, to occupational or leisure-time
friendships and pet enmities, and many others. Among them,
attachments with a sexual character between one man and one
woman certainly hold a central position in the more advanced
industrial societies. But present theoretical concepts seem to me
too narrowly connected, as I have already said, with the ideal of
marital monogamy. It might be more in keeping with the actual
observations of human beings if one allows for the fact that the
strivings of human beings towards each other and the attachments they form with each other are numerous and varied, they
have a 'group' character, not only a one man/one woman charac-

ter, even in early childhood. The term 'configuration of valencies' may be found suitable for the diagnosis and exploration of the crucial question as to how the personal configuration of valencies of each individual fits into the structure of the actual configurations he is bound to form with others in accordance with the structure and dynamics of what is currently called society at large.

The development of group psychotherapy is a good example of the way in which a therapeutic technique of great promise can suffer from the drag of a powerful professional and theoretical tradition. With very few exceptions, the theoretical framework used in the practice of group therapy is based on an individual-centred theoretical framework which makes no allowance for the differences between the structure of groups, of the configurations that individuals form with each other, and the personality structure of individuals, and which therefore does not permit a clear formulation of the problem I have just mentioned, namely how these two types of structure – structures of groups or societies formed by individuals, and structures of individuals seen singly – connect with each other. I personally know only one approach to group psychotherapy which in theory and practice is based on a clear perception of this fundamental problem – the group-analytic approach of S. H. Foulkes. I am happy to think that in this case interdisciplinary cooperation has been possible and fruitful.

Let me add one further theoretical clarification of some substance without which my basic framework would remain incomplete. One of the ways in which one tries to conceptualize the relationship of 'individual' and 'society' is that of a part/whole relationship. It is certainly not incorrect. People form part of groups. It is not unjustified to think that an individual member of a profession is a part-unit of a larger unit which he forms together with many other individuals; one can consider a nation comprising a great number of individual people as the whole, of which these individuals form part-units; and the same might be said of every other group in respect of its members. But although this conceptualization at first glance appears quite fitting, on closer examination it does not prove wholly satisfactory. If it is the aim to make conceptual models fit the evidence as closely as possible, this use of the part/whole model will have to be amended. Perhaps the simplest demonstration of its inadequacy is the relationship between the language of a society and that of one of its individual members. The individual person does not only speak part of his country's language, he assimilates and speaks the whole of the core of that language. The extent of the vocabulary may differ from individual to individual. By making allowance for variations of dialect, accent, pronunciation, and other, one can, in principle, reconstruct from the language of a single individual the whole core of the language of his society.

Nor is this the only case in which an individual embodies and represents as a kind of microcosm the whole of the social macrocosm. Thus, within the limits of his particular specialism, each member of an occupation represents in his individual person his calling as a whole. An individual judge through absorption of a judge's knowledge and long performance of a judge's work may assume the personal characteristics of a judge and at the same time represent the judge's professional characteristics as a highly distinct individual person. In the same way, an Englishman, a Russian, or an American, may show highly pronounced individual characteristics which clearly distinguish him from any of his fellow countrymen, and may, at the same time, particularly if seen together with members of other nations, be clearly recognizable as an Englishman, a Russian, or an American, and, if compared with compatriots of different classes also, as a member of a managerial, professional, or manual working class, as the case may be. Thus an individual is not only part of a whole in the same sense in which a planet forms part of a configuration of planets or an organ forms part of an organism. A human being is in some respects with his whole person representative of the whole groups or configurations that he formed or forms with other persons, while he is at the same time wholly distinct and different from all other persons.

At the present stage of sociological thinking one might be inclined to interpret such correspondences between individual and social structures simply by reference to the socialization of the individual. Although this concept is usually applied only to children and young people, it would not be out of place if one tried to extend its use. Experiences made by human beings early in life undoubtedly have a more profound influence on the developing personality structure than those made in later life. But that does not mean that later experiences have no influence at all on the personality development. Not only nursery experiences, but also experiences of a person made at school and university, and later, at work and at leisure, as parent and grandparent, in retirement and old age, go into the making of a person. As he passes through group after group he undergoes changes in his individuality. In that sense socialization never ceases as long as a person is alive.

However, the present conceptualization of the socialization of the individual, in which an individual on his passage through the various groups which he forms with others learns to live with others, is, in some respects, misleading. As it is used today, it often gives the impression that a grouping of individuals under the code name 'society' as the active agent fashions human beings singly like pieces of clay. In its present form, the concept of the socialization of the individual still reflects basic assumptions according to which a human being under the code name 'the individual' appears as an entity outside and apart from the fashioning agency of society.

It may help to restore the balance and to bring one's mode of thinking into closer correspondence with the observable evidence if one pays equal attention to another aspect of the same process, namely, to the 'individualization of social phenomena'. Not only phenomena such as the common language of a society, but also the common fund of knowledge, common norms of conduct, and many other common properties of societies become properties of their individual members as they grow up, and are on their part, as in the cases of thinking, speaking, and writing, cast in a more or less highly individual mould.

There is thus some need for a terminology that indicates more clearly the specific character of the relationship between the two aspects of men to which we refer as society and as individual, between the configurations formed by human beings with each other and the human beings in these configurations seen singly. The uniqueness of this relationship demands unique theoretical models and concepts. It may help, as an experiment, to revive for this purpose the terms 'microcosm' and 'macrocosm'. Only their application to problems of empirical research, particularly in the area linking psychology and sociology, can show whether and how far they can be developed into useful theoretical tools. They point in the right direction if they can be cleansed of their magical and mystical associations.

In the past, they were used to express the unique and mysterious correspondences between the small world of men and the large world of heaven and earth. There is nothing mysterious about the correspondences one can observe between the small world of the single human being and the large world of the configurations that human beings form with each other, as for instance correspondences between the social phenomena of a judge's profession and the characteristics of an individual judge, between English society and an individual Englishman, or between the type of social structure with high suicide rates to which sociologists apply the term 'anomie' and the personality structure that psychiatrists diagnose as suicidal tendencies, and many other correspondences of this type. At present they are often studied with the expectation that one can find complete answers in terms of a simple type of physical causality, which one might call billiard-ball causality – in terms of single-line cause-and-effect connections. But the type of connection between structures of a single human being and structures of the group he forms with others does not fit into the mould of simple causal concepts of that kind. The microcosm / macrocosm simile may make it easier in the exploration of the relationship between individual and society to go beyond the use of a billiard-ball causality concept and its derivatives.

The genuineness of an individual's self-image which expresses itself in our traditional conceptualizations is not in doubt. That the experience of oneself as a *Homo clausus* finds wide expression in the literature, in a long series of philosophical doctrines including existentialism and phenomenology, that it helps to shape theoretical assumptions in fields such as psychology and sociology, points to its representative social character. The self-awareness of a person as an isolated individual, as 'I without you', evidently is not an isolated phenomenon; it is a personal and at the same time a social phenomenon characteristic of a particular period and time.

A critical exploration of this concept of men, which underlies one's perception of human beings including oneself, requires a higher degree of self-distancing. The series of pronouns as an elementary model of a person's interdependence with others serves this function. It is not difficult to perceive that the various positions in relation to a speaker, indicated by the series of personal pronouns and used by him in his communication with others, are inseparable and interdependent. If one follows the development of a child one can sometimes directly observe how the child's awareness of himself as a separate person and his awareness of the mother, or whoever it may be, as a person separated from him, go hand in hand. One cannot say 'I' to oneself without implying 'not-you', just as one cannot say 'you' to others without implying 'you, not-I'. One can see here once more why it is not possible to use as point of departure for a study of human beings alone 'the individual' – man in the singular. It is hardly more than a truism to say that without the existence of a group of human beings no person could learn to speak or to think of himself as an 'I'.

The concept of interaction between one person and another, which is at present widely regarded as the concept of the basic type of relationship between human beings, thus, at best, scratches the surface of the relatedness of human beings. The prototype of man at the root of it is still the isolated, single individual who meets, as it were, accidentally, in the vastness of the world another individual, and then begins to interact with him. This interaction concept, too, owes its central position in present-day thinking to the perspective of adults who have lost sight of their own and of other people's development from a child, who proceed in their reflections about human beings as if they had all been born as adults, and who see themselves from within their armour as single individuals interacting with other adults equally armoured.

The relatedness of men with each other is more fundamental: it begins with being born. Underlying all intended interactions of human beings is their unintended interdependence.

NOTES

1. A more extensive discussion of these problems can be found in Elias (1969a), especially Vol. I, pp. lxii ff. and Vol. II, pp. 312 ff.
2. More recent examples of the traditional self-experience of man as a *Homo clausus* can be found in Sir John Eccles's lecture 'The experiencing self' (1969), especially pp. 105 ff. There, for example, 'But no matter how intimate is our linkage with some dearly-beloved person, we still remain separated in a most heart-rending way . . . Never does there seem to be a direct communication of one conscious self to the other.' Even the simple fact that one's language is learned from others is lost upon learned men in the bitterness of their feeling as isolated and closed systems.

3. For observations on different social patterns of love relations, see Elias, 1969b, Chapter VII, 11, p. 380.
4. The distinction between the first-person perspective and the third-person perspective – leaving aside the second-person perspective which in this context does not concern us directly – facilitates the conceptualization of some basic aspects of psychoanalytic and all related forms of psychotherapy. To put it at its simplest: The therapist tries to capture and to understand the patient's own experience connected with whatever are regarded as symptoms of mental difficulties or illnesses. He tries at one moment to see them with the eyes of the patient himself, that is, from the first-person perspective; and to perceive and interpret them at the next moment, and often enough almost simultaneously, as something that is happening to HIM or HER, that is, from the third-person perspective. By changing his position again and again from the exploration of the patient's I-perspective to the exploration of what it implies when seen from the HE-perspective, and by communicating this double perspective to the patient, the psychotherapist tries to help the patient to distance himself from the uncontrolled spontaneity of this I-experience and to perceive what he has so far experienced merely from the spontaneous first-person perspective more and more as it can be experienced by others in his society, who are here represented by the doctor proceeding in the light of his theoretical framework and the implied evaluations.

REFERENCES

ECCLES, SIR J. C. (1969). The experiencing self. In J. D. Roslansky (ed.), *The uniqueness of man*. Amsterdam and London.
ELIAS, N. (1969a). *Über den Prozess der Zivilisation*. Second edn. Bern and Munich: A. Francke Verlag.
—— (1969b). *Die Höfische Gesellschaft*. Soziologische Texte No. 54. Neuwied and Berlin.
—— & SCOTSON J. L. (1965). *The established and the outsiders*. London: Frank Cass.
HALLIDAY, J. L. (1948). *Psychosocial medicine*. New York: Norton; London: Heinemann, 1949.

8 The Study of Social Behaviour in Sub-human Primates

M. R. A. CHANCE

INTRODUCTION

The observation and recording of patterns of events without experimental interference is typical of all sciences at their inception. We may ask, therefore, why ethological studies, which are based on this procedure, have not previously taken their proper place at the base of that field of research which is collectively known as the behavioural sciences. In part, this is so because much of the tradition is concerned with the description of our own behaviour, so that traditional terms and their connotation continue to guide research and prevent our becoming aware that behaviour has structure.

Further, the prevalent view that biological phenomena are explained only in terms of their physico-chemical elements pre-supposes that they derive no properties from the intrinsic organization of their identifiable parts. Hence this view focuses attention on the constituent elements, and the organized structure of behaviour is ignored. Indeed, the restrictions of laboratory experiments seldom give an opportunity for an animal to display more than one or two elements in this structure. Hence, also, the slow progress in understanding behaviour. Sub-human primates living in their natural environment provide examples of communities living in unrestricted conditions which have recently been the subject of study by a number of vigorous and enterprising investigators. They have gone out to Africa, India, Siam, and the Gulf of Mexico to try to understand, by direct observation and recording of what they have seen, the behaviour of the members of these free-living communities. They have been ecologists, zoologists, psychologists, and anthropologists, and the different ways in which they have approached the same problem have led them to record many different aspects of these societies. An examination of their findings, as well as their mode of attack on the problem, can help us to elucidate the principles of this type of work.

This not only is necessary to assist further studies but is required in order to understand how this branch of biology should, but does not yet, include man's own behaviour. Only when this is so will a much-needed biological basis for understanding our own behaviour be achieved. As Zuckerman (1963) has put it:

> 'The attention paid by sociologists to the behaviour of the sub-human primate calls for an examination of the principles underlying comparisons between human and animal behaviour. This, in its turn, raises the further problem of defining the procedure for the development of a science of mammalian sociology.'

Carpenter (1942b) points out that it is difficult to make comparisons with human society as we know it at present because there is no appropriate and adequately specialized language. Comparisons involving human social behaviour will not be possible until the problem of *defining a procedure* for the development of a science of mammalian social behaviour is solved; therefore this article is intended as a contribution to this problem, to provide a theoretical framework which is intended to be both heuristic and explanatory.

METHOD

Each period of scientific investigation is characterized by a general conceptual system (Harré, 1964). One of these has been the attempt to explain behaviour in functional terms; thus social behaviour has been ascribed to one or more motives of the individual, leading members of a society to seek association for sexual satisfaction, mutual defence, or collaboration in hunting, etc. Apart from the fact that these concepts include different categories of explanation (because sexual satisfaction is an end-state of an individual's behaviour, defence is a state of survival, and collaboration a complex interaction between individuals), one of the chief contributions of recent ethological studies has been to eschew functional explanations until sufficient of the structure of behaviour has been revealed for us to be able to assess what are the end-states of behaviour. This has made it possible to see that one part of behaviour – a single act or recognizable signal – can have more than one function, and that parts of behaviour at present regarded for functional reasons as separate nevertheless have interactions the significance of which has so far escaped us. It can also then be seen how the parts of behaviour contribute to survival differently in different circumstances. Hence, by rigorously excluding the functional import of the terms used to describe behaviour, it may be possible to derive a new and more general conceptual system for behaviour studies.

Behaviour is what is seen of an animal's acts and postures and of its interaction through these with the physical environment or with other living things. But seeing is also selecting, and the way we select fundamentally directs the way in which the investigation is pursued.

What are the rules by which the process of selective seeing becomes the starting-point for a scientific investigation? A science begins when we first of all restrict our attention and then define the limits of the region within which we seek to elucidate the operation of the constituent parts. This process was aptly called 'the formation of an isolate' by Hyman Levy (1947). He points out that:

'Scientific truth is not an idealized truth to which the universe closely approximates, but is a *first step* in the process of finding out the truth about the universe by *examining it in chips*.'

The process of isolation has two aspects: the practical sphere of operation, within which attention is restricted, and theoretical isolates or concepts which are used to identify the whole or constituent parts of the practical isolate. As Levy again puts it:

'Science sets out in the first instance to search for systems that can be imagined as isolated from their setting in the universe without appreciably disturbing their structure and the process they present. . . .'

An isolate is, in fact, any part of the universe examined separately from its surroundings or separated physically in some way for the purposes of study. Levy points out, however, that the choice of a correct isolate is important because, if correctly chosen, it will include a stable system.

We cannot know from the start of an investigation whether an isolate has been correctly chosen. Usually it is not by virtue of our ignorance of the nature of the problem, but we are here discussing the factors which assist a good guess at the correct isolate. An isolate is only a tool of investigation, holding the problem for our inspection, and may be appropriate to only one aspect of the system under investigation. Isolates must only be used temporarily to fix our attention for just as long as it is necessary to reveal all the relevant features of the aspect we have chosen to look at. They must not be allowed to dominate our attention. Essentially, recognition of isolate formation is an instruction on how to start thinking about a scientific problem or it can be looked at as a way of relating one's thoughts to the relevant aspect of nature. Only when it is correctly fitted on to nature does it correspond to an aspect of that which we want to investigate.

It is important to realize from the start that the process of isolate formation is essentially that of defining the restriction of attention. The practical aspect of achieving this restriction of attention requires different devices for keeping the system we have under examination in view. Astronomers started in this way by confining their attention to the planets, the sun, and the moon, and isolating them for examination from all other celestial bodies, because these all moved against the background of the fixed stars. Later, as the order within this part of the system had been revealed, the isolate was increased to include our galaxy and beyond – and so astronomy came into being. The practical requirement of this work was a form of instrumentation – the telescope. By contrast, a bell jar containing a sample of gas, from which Boyle and Charles derived their laws, was a form of instrumentation which enabled them to control their system, but astronomers had no control over their isolate. Experimental control is not, therefore, an essential part of the process of abstraction which leads to the formation of scientific hypotheses or to their validation, for this is provided by the second aspect of isolate formation, the selection of adequate concepts and the construction of an adequate framework of thought. This must go hand in hand with the acquisition of facts. This integration of fact and theory is well stated by Paul Weiss (1958). He says that concepts are:

'the structural elements of a growing body of knowledge. Until distilled and ordered into concepts, data remain but a pile of incoherent information and ideas. Concepts in need of verification and consolidation guide the search for new data, and new data in turn act as tests – and, failing validation, as modifiers, of existing concepts. Thus, concepts and data must try to stay abreast.'

Naturalists have been looking at behaviour in the wild for quite a while, but reporting their findings in ways which, if vivid, have often been difficult for many scientists to believe. Putting aside credibility, however, their observations have been too widely scattered for them to have been able to establish a framework of reference by which their observations could be judged. In fact, they failed to form an isolate, and thus have not built up a science, though their observations have frequently been a starting-point for other types of systematic investigation. Ethologists are naturalists who have begun systematic observations of behaviour and have continued to watch the behaviour shown by an animal in the same situation – the nest site, the leck, etc., where usually the same natural social groups recur seasonally – thus taking advantage of natural isolates. Isolates have then been constructed in artificial circumstances: in the laboratory tank of fish or cage of birds, for example, to facilitate detailed observation either where this is difficult in the wild or when it has not been possible to find sufficient resources to spend enough time watching the wild animal. Ethologists have paid particular attention to social behaviour, in which animals are usually very active and information comes readily to hand.

THE RANK-ORDER BOND

Observation of social behaviour of mammals in the wild has been, and is being, most actively pursued in the study of the social behaviour of sub-human primates, both by moving into their territory to observe them in the wild and by imposing on them certain forms of constraint, by which observation of the behaviour within a group is made easier. Observers in the wild use instruments or place themselves in strategic positions. Semi-captive colonies are obtained by physical isolation on islands or peninsulas, and captive colonies by transferring to enclosures where there is sufficient room to allow freedom of movement. In a group of wild monkeys or apes a number of animals of different sizes and types, and of both sexes, are seen generally spread out and apparently moving about in complex fashion. But complexity itself is not a bar to the development of science; indeed, at times, as with modern physics, a deepening analysis increases the complexity. In some quarters, however, the apparent complexity of the behaviour of individuals within a group is an argument against starting an investigation of social behaviour by observing social groups; on the other hand, anthropologists have observed groups, but without a systematic attempt to overcome the limitations to their observations and way of recording them set by a conventional conceptual framework. Hence there is an urgent heuristic need to clarify the theoretical foundations upon which group behaviour can be systematically observed and the results of diverse studies correlated.

Among the studies which have already contributed to our knowledge of sub-human primate societies, Carpenter's (1934, 1935, 1940, 1942a) were the first of a series of systematic studies carried out in the wild. Carpenter realized that 'the fashions of science since about 1900 have so strongly favoured ever-increasing laboratory control that there has been serious neglect in applying the scientific method to field studies of animals, particularly monkeys and apes, man's closest phylogenetic relatives'. By this, he implicitly realized the possibilities of simple observation. He continues:

> 'The standards of scientific research which apply to laboratory investigations *can* be applied to field studies. Absolute objectivity, accuracy of recording and report and adequate samplings of observation can be made to characterize alike field investigations and those of the laboratory. The field worker, like his colleague in the laboratory, can systematically organize his data within a framework of reference which permits comprehensive description, measurement, interpretation and even prediction.'

His studies amply confirm the feasibility of his claims, but neither he nor Zuckerman has followed up their original insight into the need for a theoretical framework adequate to the tasks they foresaw. This is an attempt to take the problem a stage further.

After spending some time in the neighbourhood of a group of

monkeys, the observer can distinguish a number of different types of individual. Some of these, of course, are obvious, such as children and their mothers, but it does not take long for an observer who allows his mind to rest upon what he sees to become aware of distinctions among the adults, and later even to be able to recognize individually as many as forty different animals in a colony. Furthermore, the movement, which at first glance was no more than a set of overlapping events, soon takes on a consistency of its own, and some animals are seen to spend more time associating with another individual or with special sections of the community. In this way, spatially distinct sub-groups, which move as units in relation to other sub-groups, are seen, and they may also have distinguishing characteristics. In this way also, the intrinsic regularity, temporal as well as spatial, begins to impose itself on what the observer sees.

Carpenter frequently reported what he saw in the way a naturalist would have done. He thus established the cycle of activities within the group, during which periods of feeding, resting, and playing were clearly distinguished, and he was able to show that neighbouring groups occupied and defended territories which, on occasion, were overlapped by the feeding range. However, after he had discovered that there were two kinds of group, the heterosexual group and occasional isolated males or bachelor bands, he restricted his attention more to the heterosexual groups and finally formulated a model for the description of the group based on the identification of different sub-groups and the average spatial distances separating individuals from one another within and between these groups.

Starting, therefore, from a frankly functional and naturalistic description, he came down to a model based on intrasocial distinctions and spatial arrangements. He says:

'An important clue to social relations in primate societies is the observed spatial relations of the individuals, sub-groups and organized groups. The strength of the attachment between two individuals may be judged, or actually measured, by observing for a period of time the average distance which separates the two animals.'

In addition, he distinguished between what he calls social coordination in primate groups and group integration. This distinction is important and will be emphasized, and the meaning of the latter expanded.

Once sub-groups and typical spatial arrangements have been clearly distinguished, the problem now becomes: what are the types of interaction to be found in a society of this type? More specifically, this means: what interactions occur between the easily distinguishable sub-categories?

Unfortunately, instead of attempting to do this, and thereby drawing attention to the predominant types of interaction, he proceeds to list a number of *ad hoc* categories which are semantically noncomparable because he fails to derive the categories directly from observation and thus includes aspects other than those which are the constituent parts of the group. This error we find repeatedly in all subsequent work.

Carpenter notes that the number of possible paired interactions is given by $\dfrac{N(N-1)}{2} = 156$ for a colony of eighteen, but immediately points out that he considered only eleven categories. These are: (1) Adult males (of organized groups), (2) adult females (of organized groups), (3) adult males/adult females, (4) adult males, (5) adult females (with young), (6) young between themselves, (7) intergroups, (8) solitary or transitional animals, (9) other species, (10) ecology and climate, (11) relationship of individuals to whole group. It is difficult to see how he arrives at this selection, except by using categories traditionally accepted by sociologists or ecologists.

If, instead of imposing distinctions drawn from traditional sources on what one sees, one allows oneself to absorb and eventually become aware of the most prominent features, one is led directly to his final form of description – the prominence of certain types of association and the spatial relations.

One is soon aware, as I was, looking at the colony of Indian *Macaca mulatta* in the London Zoological Gardens, of the cohesion of the adult animals. Later it became clear that this cohesive group was prominent because, for a large proportion of the time, the constituent members were in each other's company and a high proportion of the individual's behaviour was directed towards others within the group. As I became familiar with it, the cohesion of the adult males stood out even against a background of the other members of the adult group, and I was at once struck by the fact that this cohesion might, *ipso facto*, contain the core of the social bonds keeping the society together. I shall return to this. By the same criterion, groups of females with young stood out. Careful observation shows that these consist predominantly of many mothers with their young and occasional adolescent females showing a great interest in the young ones. Finally, grooming pairs, occasional pairs of females associated together, and one or two persistently isolated individuals are also, by this token, persistent sub-divisions.

Carpenter has defined the same sub-group composition and spatial model of sub-human primate society developed directly from his observation as is suggested here as the model for starting the analysis of group structure. It is deliberately uncomplicated by refusing to construct interpretational schemes at an early stage.

Periodically, striking forms of social behaviour involving quite large numbers of individuals in agonistic interactions are seen. Interactions of this kind, whether agonistic or otherwise, may be termed 'episodes', since the interactions persist for sufficiently long to enable detailed analysis to be possible.

This raises the question: what are the types of social interaction? It cannot be assumed, as Carpenter does, that all the interactions are between only two individuals (dyadic type), or an individual and the 'rest of the colony' – whatever that means! Indeed, one of the most significant discoveries is that 'episodes' involving three or more individuals (triadic type) taking distinct forms are frequent and, in some instances, persist for a considerable time. Kummer's (in press) observations have led him to recognize triadic relations as an integral part of Hamadryas baboon society.

Carpenter's second mode of interpretation, namely that the interaction patterns should be analysed into dyadic units, must, therefore, be rejected, for he seems to be using a model derived from human society, in which one individual talking communicates to another and may, as in a lecture, talk to a large number.

Kummer and Kurt (1963) specified three ways in which the existence of sub-groups in large associations can become clear:

1. Through the spatial distribution of individuals.
2. In the frequency and types of social behaviour among the

members differing from their contacts with other individuals of the association.

3. In the time for which these two conditions persist.

Carpenter (1934, 1935, 1942a) identified the heterosexual group as the largest component of the naturally living Howler, Spider, and macaque monkeys. He also observed bands of male Howler monkeys. Together with the solitary males encountered in the Howler, Spider, Indian, and Japanese macaques, these account for some of the displaced males from observations, but the interesting case of the Takasakiyama group of Japanese macaques (Sugiyama, 1960) seems to suggest that this number is not exceeded whatever the size of the group. For between the years 1952 and 1958 the group, originally comprising about two hundred monkeys, increased to over five hundred and fifty without any increase in the number of core males. Furthermore, when at the late stage one of the core males disappeared, the remaining five still controlled the breeding hierarchy. Of half-a-dozen rather smaller groups of the Japanese macaque, the same can be said. It would seem, therefore, worth noting in future investigations whether the number of core males ever exceeds six.

Excluded males form another male association seen in the bachelor bands of Howlers and macaques, for in these societies the heterosexual group exists separately from the bachelor bands, consisting of males of equivalent age and status to the sub-dominant males of the Japanese macaque, together with an occasional excluded adult male.

The studies which have just been discussed have been available in the literature for some time and, with the notable exception of the Gibbon and probably also the savannah baboon, all show a preponderance of females in heterosexual groups and exclusion of some adult males, and all define a central rank order of males. Mainly on account of the hypothesis that sexual attraction was the bond keeping societies of monkeys and apes together, these features of the societies have been attributed to competition for mates, with the expected consequence of a high level of agonistic behaviour between males. This clearly functionally defined origin of the relationships between the adult males has, in fact, obscured the true relationships which would have emerged on the basis of observation and description of the intrinsic relations.

The rest of the article consists of a detailed examination of more recent studies in order to see whether the intrinsic relations can be discerned.

Another pair of observers to obtain information about the cohesion of sub-groups and their spatial distribution are V. and F. Reynolds (1965), who studied the chimpanzees of the Budongo forest in Uganda. They found a comparable cohesion between the males of the society. The prominence of the sub-groups is part of the Reynoldses' observations on the chimpanzee. They note at one place:

'On most days a band of from *two to five adult males* arrived after the females from an easterly direction, fed in the adjoining trees and moved on westwards toward a large group feeding about one half mile to the west.'

Or a group is recognized in different places:

'When an individual or small band was sufficiently familiar to us as to be easily recognized, it was possible to record changes in the groups associated with it. For example, one small band of *four adult males* was seen many times and seemed to be a relatively stable unit. These males were easy to distinguish both physically and behaviourally as a group (singly it would not have been possible to identify them for certain). Three were large grey-backed males. One was small and thin but also grey-backed. A fifth adult male was sometimes with them: he was old, with some white hairs, and was bald-headed.'

This band of four males was seen several times by the Reynoldses, feeding together in Maesopsis trees apart from the other bands, which would be up to half-a-mile away. Several times they were seen together with large aggregations, including mothers, juveniles, and other adults, or they would be joined by one or two adults or oestrus females who would depart before any of the others, the males of the group leaving, within minutes of each other, a site where they had been together grooming or feeding. On frequent occasions they were seen in company with each other crossing the tracks which went through the forest.

The Reynoldses says: 'The preceding examples serve to show

the way in which chimpanzee groups change and merge and indicate some of the possible bonds . . .' and they conclude:

> 'Although the composition of bands is unstable, certain *types* of grouping were frequent and may reflect an inherent structure of the social organization. The frequent types of composition were: (1) adult bands containing adults of both sexes, and occasionally adolescents, but not including any mothers with dependent young; (2) male bands containing only adult males; (3) mother bands, containing only mothers with young and occasionally other females; (4) mixed bands, containing mothers with young, other females, adolescents and adult males.'

A sub-group is, therefore, distinguished, not only by the proximity of its members and by the fact that they move from place to place in each other's company, but also, in a closely knit society, by the length of time they spend together. On the other hand, in a more loosely knit society, seen occasionally in the wild, such as the Reynoldses describe for the chimpanzees of the Budongo forest, the cohesiveness of the sub-group, such as the males, is inferred from repeated encounters with the same group recognized as a unit. They are seen in different circumstances as a separated group which occasionally intermingles with other groups at feeding-sites. One of its members may leave to associate with a member of the opposite sex, and possibly also with a group of which she is a member, but is later found back with the original group. Similarly, a male may transfer to a heterosexual group.

The studies of the Japanese macaque by Itani and Imanishi (1954, 1957) show a spatial distribution of component sub-groups. These are essentially the same as those referred to by Carpenter, and, in addition, the occasional association with a group of one or two otherwise solitary males which, from Carpenter's observations of the Howler monkey and the Gibbon, are absorbed into a group other than that from which they came. By attracting a female away from another group, they may become the primordium of a new group. The formation of a new group can also happen by subordinate males splitting off with associated females from a group.

The sub-group consisting of adult males appears in a special way in the Japanese macaque, where its separate existence has been observed not only from the features of a group, as already outlined for the chimpanzees, but from its occupation of feeding-sites where food is thrown on to open ground. The males of such a sub-group enter and are accompanied, while feeding, by the females of the society and are the first to leave it. Only when the dominant males have left do the sub-dominant and sub-adult males move in to feed. When any dominant male is present, any remaining associated females drive away the sub-dominant males, but when the sub-dominant males occupy the site they dominate all the females present, even if a few adult consorts of the dominant males remain behind. In this succession of events, the separate components of the society are seen as separate spatial sub-groups, confirmed by this order of arrival and departure.

Hans Kummer (1957) first studied a captive colony of Hama-dryas baboons in the Zurich Zoo, and later went to Abyssinia to study them in their natural habitat. He uses the same spatial criteria to identify social bonds, for he says:

'The existence of sub-groups in a large association of animals can become clear in three ways: (1) in the spatial distribution of the animals, (2) in the frequencies and types of social behaviour among the members, (3) in the time for which these two conditions persist.'

The term 'spatial coherence' is used by him in his study of the wild Hamadryas baboon to indicate that those animals in a sub-group are found closer to each other than they are to other members of the society on a high proportion of occasions. For example, he says:

'To obtain a measure of the group's coherence, we estimated the distance kept by the females from their male every five minutes during the period of observation. Using as a scale the known size of the sitting male, this is possible, with a maximum error of about 15%. From ten adult females, we obtained a total of 256 estimates, from which the mean distances could be found as 0·65 (±0·04) metres' (Kummer & Kurt, 1963).

The second feature of a sub-group he mentions is that 'significance is found in the high frequency of social intercourse among members'. It emphasizes the high proportion of attention they give to their partners in a sub-group.

His third criterion is of the persistence of groups. Two of them were observed for 103 and 124 days respectively, without any significant change in their structure. The mean period of observation per group for eight groups was sixty-one days, and in this period the number of original members only increased by two new-borns. Only one member, a sub-adult female, disappeared. Kummer mentions that the sub-groups met all his three criteria.

Kummer's studies of the wild Hamadryas baboon show that the adult breeding male is still the central figure of the community, but the special requirements of the terrain where the species lives in Abyssinia mean that they have to forage over a wide area. The social unit is the dominant male, his consort female or females, their children, and occasionally a sub-dominant male, each of which forages and moves to the nearest sleeping-place independently. This unit is recognized both in the wild and in captivity by the persistent proximity of its members and, especially in the wild, by the movement of the members of each unit as a group over large distances during the daily movements to the feeding-sites. These units come close to one another at feeding-sites, in trees, and at night, but in no place does there appear to be any interaction between adult members of adjoining units, though at water sites threats and attacks occur between the central adult males or alpha males of neighbouring units. The trees on which they feed and in which they might be expected to sleep are too small to accommodate more than a few animals at a time. Hence they become adapted to sleeping on the ledges of small cliffs some 20–30 metres high. As these are widely separated, a social unit of baboons may be caught at dusk too far from its original sleeping-quarters and so it habitually moves to the nearest cliff. This means that a 'troop', which is made up of a number of social units, encountered at dawn or dusk does not have the same composition from night to night.

It is clear that male baboons are, of all sub-human primates, best equipped with large canines, and that these are used as an effective weapon of defence against predators. Associated with this aggressive means of defence, there is a high level of overt threat and agonistic behaviour within groups of all the baboon species except the Hamadryas. It would not have been surprising to find K. R. L. Hall and Irven DeVore (1965) emphasizing in their study of the savannah baboons the aspect of overt threat in their attempts to characterize the rank-order relations between the dominant males that are prominent, and have been designated by them the 'central hierarchy'. But, in fact, they have chosen to attempt to work out the dominance pattern by importing methods from experimental psychology, which are not easily applied in the circumstances and which, in fact, proved inadequate. These essentially concentrate attention on competitive behaviour:

> 'In trying to work out the dominance pattern in the S.R. group, several criteria were used, including (1) success in achieving food objectives in paired tests given when other males were too far away to interfere directly; (2) frequency of successful dominance assertions in "natural" situations arising within a group – for example, success in gaining and maintaining access to an oestrus female, or in causing another male to move away from a particular resting place or feeding spot; (3) success of combinations of males against other individual males.'

Their difficulties begin, as they say, when they attempt linear ranking for males by these traditional criteria, for they say that other criteria, such as mounting between males, confirm the positions of top and bottom animals in the hierarchy, but do not clarify the positions of all six, partly because three of the central hierarchy males were never competitive among themselves for food although, since only one can consort with an oestrus female, they were more so over females.

Associated with this relative uncompetitiveness was the fact that they combined against other males. Linear dominance therefore does not equate with the support they get from the other males, partly because two males may dominate the group by their concerted action towards the rest. They then go on to say that, in contrast to the individual dominance status, the most significant aspect of the dominance relations in this group was that the central hierarchy males stayed together in the centre of the group.

One can sense here the tug of divergent ways of interpreting what they saw, so that they put side by side different, and apparently conflicting, aspects of the behaviour. If, instead of being concerned with the individual relationships and a hypothetical linear rank order, they noted what they saw, then the statement that 'it became clear that certain of the adult males constantly associated with each other' at the centre of the group is the starting-point of their observations, because it is the feature

M

which, on the basis of observation, isolates itself from all the rest. This single feature characterizes the behaviour of *all* the animals of this dominant group and provides the context within which the idiosyncrasies of the separate individuals give a place to the individuals within this group. If, in fact, it is the attention-binding qualities of the relationship between a dominant individual and the subordinate which places the alpha male at the centre of a stable rank order or a stable group, then it is the structure of attention within this group that is of paramount importance to understand, and the relationships between the individuals will be understood by the way they orient themselves, both spatially and in dependent types of behaviour. Elsewhere, Hall and DeVore speak about various forms of aggression, of which they list four types, according to the kinds of social interaction with which each is associated. They speak of (1) redirected aggression, (2) enlisting support-threat from others, (3) simultaneous threat (where two animals simultaneously threaten), and (4) protected threat (previously described by Kummer), which is a form of enlistment used by a subordinate animal towards one more dominant while in the shadow of the overlord male. In effect, all these will be found to be based upon a single state of awareness in subordinate animals, which is that they are continuously aware of how they stand spatially and behaviourally in relation to the alpha male. This point is practically conceded in the description by Hall and DeVore of spacing within the group during times when the group is in movement, since they say:

'It is almost impossible to discover the extent to which adults other than dominant males "lead" a group in the sense of determining the route the group will take during the day range. For example, it sometimes appeared from their frontal position that one or more of the peripheral males might be initiating group movement and determining the direction the group was to take. . . . In fact, animals in the lead were probably taking a course which was habitual to the group, but might not be otherwise determining the group's behaviour. It seems more correct to say that the group as a whole is continually alert to the behaviour and location of the dominant males and that those ahead are mainly anticipating or steering with reference to these males. This is suggested by their behaviour whenever even minor disturbances from outside the group occur, and by the fact that the main body of the group occasionally changes direction, forcing the animals who had been in front to make a wide detour before rejoining the group.'

From this it can be seen that they have, in fact, recognized the organizing pattern of attention towards the dominant males but failed to follow it up in terms of its intrinsic characteristics. Instead they say that 'the dominant animal ensures stability', 'comparative peace within the group', 'protection of mothers and infants within the group and that there is a high probability that they will be fathered by the most dominant male', or that central hierarchy males 'together control access to incentives and determine group movement'.

These are loosely defined functional outcomes of what they previously described in more accurate terms and add nothing to our understanding of how these functional outcomes are achieved. The situation is really worse than this because they suppose that we really know what functional outcomes there are, when I suspect we do not.

Turning to the dominance relations among females, they say :

'The most significant general finding from the 1960 observations on this group was the extent to which female aggressiveness against other females was correlated with the frequency of mating by the alpha male with the female who was in full oestrus.'

As they then note, this was considerably affected by the close attention of the markedly dominant alpha male to one of their number and there was 'no significant correlation with the mating frequencies of the other males'. Clearly, if attention is paid to the alpha male *per se* the aggression of the other hierarchy males aroused by him will be readily redirected at his consort, as she is also at the centre of their attention.

In his book, Schaller (1963) makes it clear that the internal organization of the group is evident in the relative spatial proximity of the different classes of individuals to the dominant male. To quote:

'Thus, the spatial organization of some gorilla groups consists of a central core composed of all females and young, as well as the dominant male, surrounded by a varying number of peripheral males.'

and again: 'The spatial organization at night tended to resemble the one found during the day.'

Schaller describes the central core of the group as composed of the dominant male and all females and young. To understand the cohesiveness we must start by an accurate description of the spatial relations and the correlated attention structure. Then it should prove possible to generalize about similarities and differences within groups of different species. How does Schaller's description fit into this scheme? Clearly, his use of the term 'quite cohesive' to describe the gorilla groups is meant to indicate that over long periods of time the members of a group stick together. He notes, for example, that the group rarely exceeds 200 ft in diameter and that, except for extra males, single individuals are rarely more than 100 ft from other members of the group. What then does he mean by a 'central core'? He does not suggest that the dominant male occupies a centrally spaced position, for he notes that while the group is moving – and that is most of the time – the position of the dominant male depends on the rate of progression. He is found at the front most of the time if the group is fast moving, and nearer the centre when slow moving. 'Every animal', Schaller says, 'is attentive to the movement of others in the dense forest environment'; yet this simple, almost casual description is again found, on closer examination, to gloss over an essential distinction. For if each gorilla pays attention to those nearest himself by keeping them in view, then, at times, one part of the group will lose sight of the other and the two will tend to drift apart. Indeed, this would appear likely to happen to the peripheral and especially the visiting males. He specifically mentions that two halves of a group may separate for as long as a day. How then does this come about on many occasions, if not by the preferential attention paid to a single dominant individual? In this way the continued cohesion of the group would be assured. Indeed, the dominant male's behaviour suggests that it is designed to demand such attention, as when, by standing motionless with legs spread, he indicates his readiness to leave a nest area. When he behaves in this way, other members of the group crowd around him.

Rank-order interactions were one of the two categories most frequently noted, the other being grooming, even though both were at a very low level (0·23 times per hour of observation). Of much greater significance was the pattern of this type of inter-action within the group. Of 110 such interactions distributed over the main classes, 51 involved subordinate animals of all classes with dominant silver-backed males; half of these (26) involving females. Four-fifths of the remainder involved all except older silver-backed males with females. This interaction pattern gives a clear indication of the pattern of attention organ-ized by the agonistic relations, for it suggests a structure of attention directly or indirectly towards the dominant silver-backed male, and would lead to the conclusion reached by Schaller on the basis of his direct observation, namely that sub-grouping in gorillas is a fairly rare phenomenon, occurring primarily in groups where more than one silver-backed male is present. In view of the large proportion of the time spent in cover it would be interesting to find out whether the calls or sounds emitted by the silver-backed are different from those of the black-backed, and whether this difference is recognized and responded to by other members of the group. Hence, if attention is focused on the dominant male, it would act as the socially integrating force, stepwise as it were, from the infants and juveniles via the females towards the black- and finally silver-backed males, one of which is the dominant member of the group. The chain of attention could then act within the group, each individual linked to the one above in his status class by the attention he pays to his immediate peer, being finally focused via the various links to the dominant male, and could naturally tend to place him nearer the front of the group during progression, the faster he himself moved. This fixation of attention of subordinate animals would then also be the mechanism by which he determines the character of the group activities. In all essential features, this is what happens in a typical baboon or macaque society. The description of the gorilla has been taken to portray an ape very different from other primates, yet the evidence here does not support the idea that the way their social integration is achieved differs in any essential way from that of some more distant catarrhine relatives.

Dominance/subordination relation in behaviour is evident in four distinct ways:

1. A subordinate will step aside from the path of a more dominant individual while on the trail.

2. A dominant will supplant another at some preferred site, such as a shady tree.

3. Rapid movement of a more dominant animal towards another will temporarily make the subordinate desist from some activity (e.g. mating), but this may be resumed later.

4. A dominant animal will bat another with its arm and thereby force it to withdraw, e.g. a female with young towards a female trying to touch her baby.

The order of dominance consists of a linear order of rank between silver-backed males in the group, if there is more than one; next, black-backed males, then females with young, females, and finally juveniles. The relationship between black-backed males and females is variable. The order of rank between females is unstable, as has been found in baboons and macaques. Size appears to determine the rank order between males, and as this is partly a function of age, the order coincides with the difference between silver-backed and black-backed. Size is also the determinant in relations between juveniles.

The dominance relations which the chain of attention postulated earlier required, are arranged stepwise.

Because the nature of Carpenter's original distinction between group integration and coordination has never been clearly appreciated, Schaller has relied on a traditional term derived from social studies of man, i.e. a 'leader' who coordinates and gives direction to human activity and 'dominance', which has been defined from the observation of animal behaviour. Hence he fails to see that, when he says that 'the dominant individual was the leader of the group', because 'any independent animal in the group appeared to be aware of the activity of the leader either directly or through the behaviour of animals in his vicinity', he is really describing the mode of operation of the social binding component of behaviour, which arises from attention directed towards him. Schaller does not in fact provide any specific evidence that 'a changed pattern of activity was patterned after the leader', referring mainly to aspects of the daily routine, such as distance of travel, location of rest stops, and time and place of nesting, all of which types of behaviour flow naturally from remaining in his vicinity and are in no way dependent on 'a change in type of his [the dominant male's] own behaviour'.

Schaller's observations are prodigious, and we put forward an alternative explanation only because it is essential (1) to recognize that current terminology may be forcing our attention into the wrong channels and (2) to emphasize the need to work out the fundamental nature of the social relations within these natural social groups. Schaller considers the relevant material under what he calls the internal organization of the group in two aspects: spatial arrangement and dominance relations, but although they show a considerable identity of pattern, Schaller does not see any link between them. Whereas, by suggesting that the cohesion of the groups is maintained by the degree of attention paid by subordinate members to those immediately dominant over them, a pattern of association emerges which exactly fits the spatial arrangement and provides also a means of understanding (1) how the spatial arrangement follows from the hierarchical relations and (2) how the secondary aspect of this is the way in which the dominant male appears to act as leader, for it can be seen that this so-called leadership does not consist of anything more than what flows directly from his attention-demanding behaviour.

Thus far, we have considered the cohesion between the members of the group. What can now be said about the tendencies of individuals to move in and out of the group?

Lone males are a distinct and important feature of the population structure. As in the populations of Indian and Japanese macaques, Howler and Spider monkeys, where lone males are also a feature, lone females were not seen.

Schaller says that the lone gorilla male associates freely with some groups, by which is meant that he wanders, apparently unmolested, through the group. On one occasion a lone silver-backed male was threatened by the dominant male of a group as he approached, and he did not advance further. It appears that lone males who attach themselves to the outer edge of the groups for one or two days are at one end of a range of what may be termed visiting males, some of which stay for as long as several months as an integral part of the group. These visitors are adults of all ages. However, it is worth noting that, out of six groups, these visiting males only associated with two.

Schaller comments on what he regards as a popular supposition, that 'lone males have been *forcibly* (our emphasis) thrown from the groups by rivals' and suggests that, because he observed 'no strife' between males in a group, 'the readiness with which they left and joined some groups suggested that they did so freely'. In our view, this is where the failure to give clear definition to the structure and processes operating to control behaviour leads an observer to fall back on the use of language wholly insufficient in scope and meaning to indicate further useful lines of observation. It is well known from studies of other social animals that rank-order relations can bring about the breaking-away of low-ranking males as the result of the inability of the latter to remain long in the presence of those more highly placed: that is to say, those to whom they defer. Their withdrawal is, in these instances, less a result of active threats directed at them and more a result of their propensity to escape from the presence of those whose more relaxed behaviour indicates a stature of assurance they do not possess.

What better confirmation of such a suggestion can one want than the statement made in another context: 'members of a group were alert to the possibility of aggressive encounters, and subordinate animals tended to circumvent the issues before they materialized'?

Fluctuations in the mood of the submissive animal could then be sufficient cause, though clearly, in actual fact, this would rarely be so, to account for the fluctuating association of such animals with the groups to which they attach themselves. This possibility, that changes in the repulsion between associates is the cause of their separation, is as important to bear in mind as is the alternative, whereby changes in their attraction for one another is a contributory cause. Such a framework at least makes the alternatives clear, and does not engender a premature satisfaction, which, on reflection, leaves one wondering what is meant by 'gorillas which join or leave the group *quite freely*'.

The purport of this paper has been to point out that the isolation and description of prominent intrinsic features of social groups leads to the discovery of a bond uniting the society and that it can be deduced that this operates through the structure of attention. This bond is capable of binding the agonistic relations within the society, though it is present when these are minimal. The method is in direct contrast to the common approach, which is illustrated by Phyllis Jay (1965a) in her chapter on 'Field studies' in *The behavior of non-human primates*, where she regards the field as a 'natural laboratory', in which

> 'learning, perception, affection, curiosity, etc., are important aspects of primate behaviour. . . . But the adaptive functions of each of these aspects of behaviour are clear only in a free-ranging social situation where the advantages of being an intelligent, perceptive, affectionate, curious animal can be seen, as they cannot be seen in a laboratory or cage.'

It is not possible to decide from Phyllis Jay's own description (1965a) of the social behaviour of the common langur of North India whether or not there is a separate spatially distinct core, comprised of the most dominant adult males, although they appear to form a stable rank order. This is because, like so many observers, her concern is as much with defining the functional outcomes of the behaviour as with the behaviour itself, and, inevitably, the two get confused. It is important, and indeed revealing, to recognize that the langur is a relatively large, lithe, long-limbed monkey, which moves with large graceful bounds which, in an emergency, take each individual adult back to the safety of nearby trees. Hence, it is in escape that safety is found. Indeed, Jay concedes the essence of the main thesis that the objective attention is the process which determines the outcome of an animal's behaviour during excitement when she says that 'they dash up into the nearest tree instead of depending for protection on large adult males with well-developed fighting prowess', but since it is couched by reference to the functional outcome, the fact that it is the direction of attention that matters escapes her notice.

Equally confusing to the further discussion of the nature of sociability is her statement that 'most of the activities which occupy an individual's time are unrelated to dominance status', for here again expression by overt forms of behaviour is the only way in which the relation of one animal to another in a rank order is assessed. This is a pity, because she comes closer than most observers to the inclusion of the necessary information by noticing that avoidance of one animal by another is at least as important in assessing rank: for example, she says,

'Reduction of all dominance interactions to numbers of successes and failures is only a partial reflection of the dominance structure, and needs qualification. Patterns of social interaction most difficult to evaluate, such as avoidance, are extremely important in understanding dominance.'

This awareness of spatial arrangement is further emphasized by her noticing that individuals have what she calls 'a personal space' surrounding them, which is, in size, related to their status. This phenomenon was first noticed by Chance (1956) in the captive colony of Indian macaques at the London Zoo, and given the name of social space.

Unfortunately, however, Jay does not follow up the logical implications of this aspect of the behaviour. This has much to contribute in explaining two aspects of the society, one of which is peculiar to this type of monkey and is not just a minor aspect of behaviour. The presence of bachelor bands in langurs (the name given to groups of males found together, separate from the rest of the society) indicates, as in other monkeys, that there is a strong bond between the males that can assert itself in the appropriate circumstances, and this appears in the ontogeny of the male (not of the female) in the approach behaviour of ten-month-old males towards the dominant males.

'At this time, the infant first approaches the adult in a highly specialized manner. The infant runs, squealing tensely, to the moving adult, and veers away just before it touches him. Gradually the infant appears to gain confidence and touches the male's hind-quarters. Within a week after this, the infant approaches and mounts by pulling himself up over the adult's hind-quarters. Infant mounting of an adult male is similar in form to a male mounting a female or to dominance mounting between two adults, but when displayed by the infant it is neither sexual nor dominance behaviour. In a few weeks, another element is added and the infant runs round to face and embrace the adult. Touching, mounting and embracing occur thereafter either as a series or as separate events. . . . The male juvenile mounts and embraces adult males more than four times as often as does the male infant of ten months old.'

Subsequent to this, the sub-adult behaviour shows that this behaviour is suppressed while it moves to the periphery of the group before taking its place in the adult community.

These two pieces of evidence suggest that the young male langur, like other primates, has a strong built-in approach tendency towards adult males which may be less easy to distinguish in the adult, and, if indeed absent, is only overlaid by the more species-specific behaviour, while the adult is part of the heterosexual group, but which does reassert itself in bachelor bands.

RANK-ORDER BOND IN CAPTIVE COLONIES

We must thank the ingenuity and careful observation of the different fieldworkers for the data that are so comparable and have yielded so consistent a picture. Their observations on a number of wild species of monkey and ape have shown that the members of one kind of group or another spend much time in each other's company, both while the group they so compose is stationary and when it moves long distances.

When a sub-group is out of sight of another one, all the social behaviour of a member of a group is clearly restricted to the other members of that group. How far, we ask, is this so if the groups come together? Kummer describes how the individuals in one social unit of the Hamadryas baboon do not have any social intercourse with members of others when they gather together at the sleeping-cliffs. Hence, we may ask, how far does this restricted social attention operate and cause the cohesion of members of a sub-group? We should ask ourselves how far this restriction of attention to members of the group, of which a baboon is a member, is the result of a continuation of the behaviour which binds the attention of the individual to a dominant male. If, when other groups are nearby, this is intensified even at the expense of attention to other members of its own group, then we shall have evidence that it is the quality of the bond between the subordinate members and the overlord male which is responsible for the cohesion of the group in all circumstances. We want to know, therefore, more about the attention that one member pays to another.

Consider more closely the relationships within the group of adult males, which are a central part of all but three of the ten species studied. The easiest way to do this is to look at a captive colony of monkeys, such as the Indian macaque, which has been established with a correct sex ratio. This is what I did at the London Zoological Gardens in 1952 (Chance, 1956), but essentially the same type of procedure as I am about to describe could be adopted to understand the bonds uniting members of such a group in any wild monkeys with which contact can be maintained for reasonably long periods of time. It is necessary to do this in the wild in order to find out what the integrating factors are which hold them together or, in other words, what is the nature of the bond which unites them. It is not really adequate merely to suggest that, for the chimpanzee, habit or friendship is a sufficient explanation, nor does the mode of their movement together suggest that they are merely following an habitual route in a fixed sequence from one fruit tree to another. Much more pertinent is the fact that a group of adult males was seen separated as a group and its members were together for long periods of time, for this must be a measure of the degree of attention they paid to each other. Indeed, I suggest that what Carpenter sees as the integrating factor in these societies is precisely the amount of attention that one animal pays to another. Further evidence of a different kind shows that this is so (see below).

The value of captive colonies is that they make possible observation of the way in which sub-groups keep together, provided that the colony has been isolated from its natural environment in an appropriate manner and has, as a result, an adequate composition and structure to be viable.

The problem of forming an appropriately constructed colony depends, therefore, on the proper assessment of what the social unit is in the wild. From what is known from Kummer's study of the wild Hamadryas baboon, it is clear that the requirements which follow from such an assessment were not met by Zuckerman's (1932) original study, for two reasons: (1) it enclosed a number of social units on Monkey Hill in the London Zoo which would not normally be brought into close contact except at night, and which are known to skirmish with each other when they meet at water holes and feeding-sites during the day; and (2) the socionomic index for this monkey, as for others, shows a preponderance of females. The fact that the males outnumbered the females on Monkey Hill aggravated the tendency for the males of the social units to fight when kept close together. The captive colony which Zuckerman studied was not, therefore, an appropriate isolate. Special features of each colony exist which it will be most instructive to unravel in the future, and these determine to some extent the character of each colony, but these idiosyncrasies need not worry us too much for our present purposes.

In the London Zoo colony of Indian macaques, established with the correct sex ratio of adults, the deflection of attention of the subordinate males of the dominant set towards the overlord or to the one next in rank was most evident. This repeated deflection of attention up the hierarchy was accompanied by submissive behaviour towards the dominant male, even when this was not evoked by any overt threat directed towards the subordinate members of the rank order. Hence their repeated glances in his direction, and submissive movements (presentation and adjustment of spatial relations), were in response to a status which they recognized in him and which may have been communicated to them constantly by his posture and the way in which the markings of his fur emphasized this posture uniquely.

Kummer makes the same point when he says of the Hamadryas baboon: 'A collation of all the protocols shows that in almost all cases an individual which is afraid will seek out the largest animal near it.' And: 'The seeking out of the high ranking animal is an elementary form of behaviour which illustrates the commanding position of the old male.'

This deflected attention, then, would be the mechanism which is associated with, or is part of, the attraction of the subordinate animals towards the dominant one, as it is met with in many different vertebrates. It is, without doubt, balanced by a certain tendency to move away from the more dominant animal, as can be seen from the fact that each male slept with his consort female separated by a few feet from the others: a spatial separation which was typical of them at rest and at other times as well. It is also evident in the typical distances which separated them at different phases of the colony.

Courting female macaques in the London Zoo were aggressive to their overlord; holding his attention in this way and in ways which we shall consider later, they were able to convert this relationship into a quieter and more stable bond. That attention is a bond-forming process can also be seen in the way in which young monkeys attract to themselves not only their own mother, but also other females with or without young. The females, after looking at them for a long time, move towards these young and attempt to play with them and lure them away from their mothers, or actively snatch them up if they are already removed to a sufficient distance from their mothers. Here they are occupied in *doing* something with another animal which attracts their attention, whereas, in the dominant set, the submissive animals are obsessively attentive towards the dominant male.

In sub-human primate societies, therefore, 'integration', as Carpenter calls it, is the result of prolonged attention spans which must, by their very nature, more or less exclude attention to other aspects of the individual's surroundings. In just what ways this divided attention results in a conflict, and what are its consequences, are aspects of the social behaviour yet to be understood. But Sutherland (1964), who has shown that the more an animal pays attention to one aspect of the environment the less it pays to others, may have provided a route into this problem. In view of the potential conflict between what Carpenter calls 'integration' and coordination based on communication, the term 'integration' should be replaced by a more appropriate description, namely 'bonding attention'.

GROOMING AS A SOCIAL BOND

Because of the emphasis placed on the existence of the rank-order bond by the methods of study advocated here, it must be emphasized that other bonds exist and are made evident by the same criteria, the next most important being grooming.

Despite the difficulties of his study, Zuckerman noticed and recorded, though possibly with insufficient emphasis for subsequent readers to pick up the points, examples that illustrate the two main bonds brought to light by other workers. These were the attachment of a subordinate male to one particular overlord, and the prominence of grooming as a social bond. For, as Zuckerman says: 'It seems very likely that the social performance of grooming . . . always remains one of the fundamental bonds holding sub-human primates together.'

This quotation from Zuckerman is borne out by the most comprehensive study of this activity which, to my knowledge, has yet been made. Reynolds (1961) found that, on average, at least 45 per cent of the time was spent in grooming by monkeys of the Whipsnade Zoo colony in the year 1960. A number of other workers, including the Japanese, agree that a large proportion of the time is spent by monkeys in this activity.

Grooming consists of searching through the fur of another animal, which adopts a suitable posture to facilitate this activity. The activity can be one-way, or mutual. Self-grooming was not included in Reynolds's study, since it does not involve an encounter between two animals. He has provided detailed quantitative information on this activity in the colony, measured by his unit of grooming activity. Each bout is recorded under the 'initiator', that is to say, the animal that starts the grooming. In this way, it has been found that the activity fluctuates in total quantity over a period of several months. It is shown by an individual after the first year, and so appears to be an adult activity, restricted mainly to the females and correlated fairly strongly with dominance. Although it is often a catholic activity, it can also be restricted to one or more partners, and, in some instances, is so restricted over a long period of time, increasing in intensity as the amount of total activity in the rest of the colony decreases.

In those partnerships which persist and are exclusive, there must be instances in which, judged by the amount of time spent with the grooming partner, this activity would constitute a bond in the sense in which it has been previously defined. In other instances, where the grooming of the initiator is with a number of different monkeys, it would be unlikely to be so. Nevertheless, such obsessive activity might bring about a more general bonding of the community through the large amount of time spent on one social activity. Without sufficient data concerning the amount of time spent in each bout, or the other activities such as following or sitting next to (defined by Reynolds), both of which could reflect the same bonding attention, which might or might not include grooming as a component part, we cannot give greater definition to this area of investigation. This discussion emphasizes the value of clarifying the criteria by which behavioural observations are made and described.

Grooming occupies an equal status with agonistic behaviour as judged by frequency and total time in the life of the gorilla, although both activities are at a very low level. Mutual grooming is, however, not practised.

Partly because of differences in methods of approach, the Reynoldses had little opportunity of observing this activity in the chimpanzee, but Jane Goodall (1965) gives some comprehensive information. Grooming may be mutual or one-way, and interesting facts are given about the frequency of grooming between the different categories of individual. It is shown that nearly half the activity is between adults, and the rest is distributed down the population according to age. In this connection it is of particular interest that a mature male is most likely to groom or to be groomed by another mature male, and the female by another mature female, and that a female in oestrus is more likely to be groomed by a male than is a non-receptive female.

Thus it appears that the fact that there are bands of adult males within which attention is directed to other members of the band may account for the preponderance of grooming between males.

In notable contrast are the grooming tendencies of the savannah baboons (studied by Hall and DeVore), which are prominent; here, the bouts between females are five times longer than bouts between males.

Insufficient evidence is given by Jay's description of grooming in the langur for much to be said about it, but it would appear to provide a bond between adult males and females, and between adult females, and between adult females and their young, but since there is virtually no grooming indicated between the sub-adult males and any other section of the community, and yet the agonistic bonds are clearly indicated, this is additional evidence that the male agonistic bond exists in langurs.

That bonding by grooming relations is an important element can be seen in societies of most species, but its full understanding would appear to require a wider scheme of reference, because the direction and intensity of this activity are so different in the different communities.

CONCLUSION

The suggestion that, at this early stage of the study of the wild societies of monkeys, more attention should be paid to theoretical formulations might seem to be premature, because at this stage collecting information about the different species would seem to be the most urgent task, in order to provide the foundations for subsequent theorizing, but at the beginning of this article it was made clear that observations involve selection, and that, since we are living in an unformulated climate of thought about what we do, we at present make false selections and miss opportunities.

Far from being a criticism of the energy and resourcefulness of all those who have gone out into the wild, it is likely that the acceptance, after discussion, of working hypotheses will facilitate the collection of data that are then capable of being correlated from a number of different species. In fact, this is the most disappointing aspect of the various reports; that they do not, in fact, provide the evidence for any far-reaching theoretical formulation, and thereby force the workers to import *ad hoc* assumptions, which are clearly not derived from the data themselves. These are often of traditional origin, imported from psychology, or are supposed functional consequences. All too often we are thus led to assert that this movement or that sound communicates something to another animal, without any objective evidence. Hence I think it is impossible to find any single unequivocal example of behaviour acquired by learning in a social context, except where it has been looked for by the Japanese workers, yet this idea is referred to in practically every study. Another omission is the lack of definition in the word 'role' to express the outcome of the individual's behaviour in the society, and a prominent example of this is the failure to define what it is in the rank-order relations that brings about the departure of low-ranking individuals from the group, despite notable concern in all the studies with this aspect of social life. Whether or not the formulation put forward here to explain this particular phenomenon is accepted in the form in which it is presented, it cannot be denied that the observations adduced in support of the suggestion that it is the idiosyncrasies of the subordinate individuals which are responsible for this, more than the nature of the overt aggressiveness of the dominant animals, at least provide a formulation with which one can discuss the bearing of the adduced evidence and ways of looking for further evidence.

The criticism of terminology that has been part of this essay has done more than draw attention to the vagueness of words, or to the fact that the use of terms of traditional origin tends to obscure from view the underlying pattern of events, for it has been possible to see that, irrespective of their origin, these terms represent a hidden dichotomy of interest in the approach these

N

observers adopt. Indeed, it appears that they are ranging over three different levels of biological organization without being aware of it. There is the discussion that tends to be satisfied with an explanation of the functional outcomes such as the achievement of safety, the exploitation of food resources, etc., which are clearly defined and are within the sphere of the adaptation of the animal to its environment. Such explanations are satisfactory in every way, provided that the behaviour can be shown to have the stated outcome. Within the society itself, this approach has led to the deflection of attention away from the most important feature, namely the structure of social relations discovered through an accurate description of grouping tendencies. The attribution of supposed functions is far less satisfactory in many instances, and is often the result of importing concepts from the laboratory, as in statements such as that the social maturation of the individual is the concern of the whole group, for they do not lead anywhere. Similarly, the statement that the monkey's life is a complex adaptation in learning to get along with others does not assist theoretical formulation; nor is the attempt to explain the social matrix by suggesting that it is a framework providing the necessary contact with age-mates for the development of a normal adult monkey (as has been demonstrated in laboratory analysis) any justification for saying that this is a reason for the existence of a stable group, within which such a process could take place. Nor can group stability be ascribed to assuming 'roles' and activities which assure group cohesion and specific inter-group relations, without imparting a cloak of semiconscious outcomes to a discussion which, in all other respects, does not attempt to provide any evidence of the degree of individual awareness of a role.

Finally, there are the explanations which are sought in terms of the physiology of the individual and which take the physiological requirements as primary and the behavioural aspects as satisfying these, rather than seeing that there is an interaction between them, the physiology being both influenced by, and itself often the pre-condition for, social behaviour.

If the existence of a society of free-ranging animals depends on the simple fact that its members remain together within this range for prolonged periods, then the strength of the bonds uniting different constituent individuals will be likewise measured by the frequent proximity of those individuals to one another. Thus because some individuals are more attracted to each other than are others, these will form sub-sections or bands within the society. A review of ten studies on ten different species of sub-human primate reveals that in no instance has this criterion been used as the foundation on which to base the description of the structure of each society, despite the initial suggestions along these lines put forward by Carpenter in 1942. This is, in part, due to the absence of adequate theoretical discussion of the problem, and hence to the carry-over of obsolete concepts which continue to encase thought on this subject. Nevertheless, sufficient evidence is presented (though in no instance has it so far been stated) to show that, in seven out of the species examined, a stable spatial relation of the adult males is the core of the society, and that this bond is dependent on a compulsive deflection of attention of subordinate males towards those high in rank or towards the supremely dominant male. Evidence exists to show that this deflection of attention appears in the development of male langurs before it disappears in the adult. If, as is contended, the deflection of a subordinate's attention is the most significant feature perpetuating rank-order relations, then the behaviour of subordinate individuals is of equal significance in understanding rank-order relations as the current view that it is the aggressive behaviour of dominant individuals which engenders rank-order relations.

Attention to another animal may not amount to anything more than awareness of a companion, even at a distance, and hence the importance or role of sounds may do no more than enable contact between separated habitual companions to be restored; e.g. chimpanzee noises, and the calls of other species. Hence the concern with social organization rather than sociability in the first instance presupposes a level of complexity which is, very probably, in the majority of instances, unjustified by the evidence. It leads Eisenberg (1966), in his recent monograph on the social organization of mammals, to list as the first of his criteria of social organization 'a complex system of communication' rather than what he places third – sociability, or, as he puts it, 'cohesion or the tendency of the members to remain together'.

The principle of this article has been to suggest that evidence for underlying sociability (Carpenter's integration) should be sought independently, and before trying to discover more complex aspects of social life, for it may be simple attention which subserves the single tendency of animals to cohere to one another. If this is directed at one dominant individual, he thereby determines group activities by bringing the subordinate individuals into situations where their attention becomes similarly oriented and thus they become responsive to the same elements that are present in their surroundings. This type of influence of a dominant individual on others of the society is much simpler than if they were to learn by imitation or else imitate an activity by example. The use of the term 'leader' to encompass these and more complex activities merely prevents progress of thought on the matter.

The behaviour of subordinate individuals suggests that for a large amount of their actual life their attention is on more dominant individuals and this is a feature extending throughout the society, so that directly, or in a stepwise fashion, the attention of all the individuals and classes of individual is focused towards the dominant male. Moreover, it then becomes clear that competition as such has nothing intrinsically to do with rank-order relations, but may accentuate them or modify their form.

It is suggested that attention fixation up a rank order towards a dominant male may be a widespread basis of primate sociability among the simian stock and may perhaps be phylogenetically very old, since it is met with in the societies of other vertebrates.

NOTE ON THE NATURE OF A SOCIAL ISOLATE IN HUMAN SOCIETIES

The attention structure that has been outlined does much to control the behaviour of individuals in a group, but a significant feature of the individual sub-human primate's social behaviour is that his social contacts are restricted to one group only. That is to say, he does not pass back and forth easily between groups whose members do not know each other. This is because, in all species except the apes, strangers are treated with hostility. Of the apes, gibbon groups threaten each other vocally across territorial boundaries, and, when the calling has died down, members of the different groups mingle for a few minutes. This behaviour is already different from that of the rest of the simian stock, and in the behaviour of gorillas towards strangers there is evidence of much reduced hostility. Some male gorillas pass into and out of groups gradually and are associated with any new group for months, or at least weeks, at a time.

Reynolds claims that chimpanzees readily enter into social relations with strangers, but evidence for this is not yet conclusive.

Human beings are, at least in modern societies, able to pass daily between communities at their place of work and back to home, in some instances stopping off less regularly but nevertheless often enough to be on familiar terms with members of a club or similar association. Likewise, the members of these separate associations have relations with yet other groups.

This difference must be borne in mind when considering the isolates made for the study of human social behaviour. A person's social environment is, therefore, not just his immediate contacts within the group in which he may be seen at any given moment, but also includes the pattern of social relations made in a number of different groups. That his behaviour in one group is influenced by the nature of his relations with other groups is therefore an important feature to include within the compass of a study relating to individual social behaviour. Methods for doing this have not been adequately worked out by either sociologists or psychologists.

This is pertinent to the problem of how effective therapeutic groups are. In them, the individual is given the opportunity to discover what his fears are and to have these fears assuaged by seeing others coping with their own. Whether or not he is able to benefit from the changes in his own ways of behaving towards others, which he may eventually achieve, will depend upon whether or not there are correlated changes in the home background or among his workmates. That is to say, whether these are permitted to occur or whether changes are actively resisted by the other members of these other groups. It would seem necessary, therefore, to promote an awareness in the members of these groups that changes may be expected, and to enlist their support in bringing them about. Contemporary social relations from other groups to which the individual belongs may fix or facilitate changes as much as do subconscious processes derived from a person's past experience.

REFERENCES

CARPENTER, C. R. (1934). A field study of the behaviour and social relations of Howler monkeys (*Alouatta palliata*). *Comp. Psychol. Monogr.* **10**, 48–168.

—— (1935). Behaviour of red Spider monkeys in Panama. *J. Mammal.* **16**, 171–80.

—— (1940). A field study in Siam of the behaviour and social relations of the Gibbon (*Hylobates lar*). *Comp. Psychol. Monogr.* **16**, 5.

—— (1942a). Sexual behaviour of free ranging Rhesus monkeys (*Macaca mulatta*). I. Specimens, procedures and behavioural characteristics at oestrus. II. Periodicity of oestrus, homosexual, autoerotic and nonconformist behaviour. *J. Comp. Psychol.* **23**, No. 1.

—— (1942b). Societies of monkeys and apes. *Biol. Symp.* **8**, 177–204.

CHANCE, M. R. A. (1956). The social structure of a colony of *Macaca mulatta*. *Brit. J. anim. Behav.* **4**, 1–13.

EISENBERG, J. F. (1966). The social organization of mammals. *Handbuch der Zoologie* **10**, No. 7, 1–92. Berlin: Walter de Gruyter.

GOODALL, J. (1965). Chimpanzees of the Gombe Stream Reserve. In I. DeVore (ed.), *Primate behavior*, pp. 425–73. New York and London: Holt, Rinehart & Winston.

HALL, K. R. L. & DEVORE, I. (1965). Baboon social behavior. In I. DeVore (ed.), *Primate behavior*, pp. 53–110. New York and London: Holt, Rinehart & Winston.

HARRÉ, R. (1964). *Matter and method.* London and New York: Macmillan.

IMANISHI, K. (1957). Social behaviour in Japanese monkeys (*Macaca fuscata*). *Psychologia* **1**, 47–54.

ITANI, J. (1954). Japanese monkeys at Takasakiyama. In K. Imanishi (ed.), *Social life of animals in Japan.* Tokyo: Kobunsya (in Japanese).

JAY, P. (1965a). Field studies. In A. M. Schrier, H. F. Harlow & F. Stollnitz (eds.), *The behavior of non-human primates*, Vol. 2. New York and London: Academic Press.

—— (1965b). The common Langur of North India. In I. DeVore (ed.), *Primate behavior*, pp. 197–249. New York and London: Holt, Rinehart & Winston.

KUMMER, H. (1957). Soziales Verhalten einer Mantelpavian-gruppe. Beiheft *Schweiz. Z. Psychol.* **33**, 1–91.

—— (in press) Tripartite relations in Hamadryas baboons.

—— & KURT, F. (1963). Social units of a free-living population of Hamadryas baboons. *Fol. Primatol.* **1**, 4–19.

LEVY, H. (1947). *The universe of science.* (Rev. edn.) London: Watts.

REYNOLDS, V. (1961). The social life of a colony of Rhesus monkeys (*Macaca mulatta*). Ph.D. Thesis, University of London.

REYNOLDS, V. & F. (1965). Chimpanzees of the Budongo forest. In I. DeVore (ed.), *Primate behavior*, pp. 368–424. New York and London: Holt, Rinehart & Winston.

SCHALLER, G. B. (1963). *The mountain gorilla: ecology and behavior.* Chicago and London: University of Chicago Press.

—— (1965). The behavior of the mountain gorilla. In I. DeVore (ed.), *Primate behavior*, pp. 324–65. New York and London: Holt, Rinehart & Winston.

SUGIYAMA, Y. (1960). On the division of a natural troop of Japanese monkeys at Takasakiyama. *Primates* **2**, No. 2.

SUTHERLAND, N. S. (1964). Visual discrimination in animals. *Brit. med. Bull.* **20**, 54.

WEISS, P. (1958). Concepts of biology. *Behav. Sci.* **3**, No. 2.

ZUCKERMAN, S. (1932). *The social life of monkeys and apes.* London: Kegan Paul.

—— (1963). Human sociology and sub-human primates. In C. H. Southwick (ed.), *Primate Social Behavior*. Princeton, N. J., and London: Van Nostrand.

9 Psychology and the Ideology of Progress

PAUL HALMOS

INTRODUCTION

Ideologies of progress sprout from an inextinguishable hope that one day things will be better. Somewhere ahead life will be more abundant and there will be less pain and fear. Somewhere ahead there will be more rationality, objectivity, and truth. Somewhere ahead there will always be more love and compassion for others (Ginsberg, 1961, pp. 1–56; Eder, 1962). Any combination of these and of other values could easily be extracted from the literature of progress. When writers begin with the thesis, 'there is progress in the realization of values', they assume two things. First, they put forward a sociological-historical hypothesis according to which social changes proceed in a set direction and fall into some sort of sequential pattern; and, second, they contrive to find that, on the whole, in this sequence, there is a linear increase in the realization of some values which they regard as essential to humanity. A careful inspection of the second of these two assumptions discloses the belief that not only things will be getting better and better but people too. Those, then, who are ideologists of progress are committed to a coherent directionality not only in the betterment of circumstances but also in the betterment of people; in brief, social changes will be accompanied by changes in the 'modal' personality as well.

In spite of the great multiplicity of accounts describing the critical values which are supposed to be increasingly realized by man in the course of his social development, one critical value seems to receive more prominent mention than any of the others. It comes in various guises, for example, as 'altruism', 'sympathetic imagination', 'capacity for identification', 'fellowship', 'cooperation', 'kindness', and of course '*love*'. Even when other neutral-sounding words are used, such as 'humanism' or 'wisdom', love is still implied but it is self-consciously concealed in less senti-mental-seeming terms, for surely neither humanism nor wisdom could be conceived as meaningful unless they included the orientation of loving as well. It is then hardly an oversimplifi-cation to say that the ideologies of progress arrange their account of history so that the chain of historical episodes can be shown to represent human behaviour of a growingly loving nature and that the series of episodes could also be plausibly extrapolated into the future in which this growth can confidently be expected to continue (Halmos, 1957, Ch. 1).

We have, therefore, before us not only a sociological hypothesis about social development but also a psychological hypothesis about the progressive development of 'modal' person-ality so that it embodies more and more readiness to behave lovingly, or, if you like, kindly, tolerantly, as well as imaginatively and sensitively. Or, to phrase it differently, human social develop-ment is of such a kind that it moulds man in its social behaviour to be more frequently, variedly, and effectively loving of other people.

One might say that the doctrine of progress is a doctrine of the growth of love, and my task is to examine what effect, if any, our psychological interpretations of the experience of love, or, if you like, of 'loving behaviour', have on the growth of love in human society.

The presence of psychology in the stream of an allegedly progressing culture must of necessity act on the culture of which it is a part. This is manifest enough from the way in which our social and moral development has been coloured by widely disseminated and popularized psychological notions and inter-pretations in the twentieth century. Few items of legislation or processes of administration of health, welfare, or education have escaped the influence of psychological appraisal. One may say that there is no new issue to be resolved here and that there is no urgent diagnosis to be made. I am, however, prompted by antici-pations of a major change in the nature of this psychological influence and the hypothesis in this paper concerns this expected change.

The hypothesis I am going to consider is suggested to me by the following considerations: as social change follows social change, the moral fibre of the period will be at least toned by the life-blood of ideas and images that happen to be circulating. In past centuries, religious and philosophical ideas inspired and regulated much of human conduct, loving and affectionate or otherwise. In the twentieth century, two major groups of psychological theories have joined the theological-philosophical interpreters and dealers of ideas about love and hate. These two I shall call, rather uninventively, *vitalistic* and *mechanistic* psychologies. As to the first of these two: during the first half of the twentieth century and even to this day the large-scale influencing of public opinion, of nursery practices, and of institutional arrangements and procedures has been guided either by traditional ethical considerations or by the notions of a vitalistic psychology which, as I will hope to show, have reinforced the traditional ethical regimens of love, sympathy, and honesty. During these decades, the mass media of communication have profusely and ubiquitously advertised psychoanalytic insight as kindness, acceptance, tolerance, and permissiveness, and have made the moral lesson taught by this and other related vitalistic psychologies indistinguishable from the moral lessons of Christianity. In the meantime, the second group of psychologies, that is the mechanistic psychologies, flourished too, but their key concepts have not spread out into the various private and public sectors of life or succeeded in making an impression on man as an experiencer of love, sympathy, or concern. Somehow, mechanistic psychology would never venture far outside the laboratory. It seems to me that since the re-emergence of Pavlovian methods in contemporary 'behaviour therapy', since the spreading application of learning theory to clinical treatment, and since the reappraisal of maternal love in terms of sensory stimulation, we may well be on the threshold of a period during which the relatively peaceful armistice-like compact between traditional ethics and psychoanalytical metaphysics may be outdated by the rude objectivity of new ideas. *My hypothesis is that to preserve its positive contribution to the growth of love in man's progress, the more objective and quantitative psychology succeeds in becoming, the more it will have to turn its attention to the psychological problems created by the impact of its own growth in articulation and precision on human behaviour.*

Before this hypothesis is examined, certain general observations should be made in respect of *all* psychological inquiry, be it vitalistic or mechanistic in its basic categories. It is common knowledge that an attempt at understanding is an attempt at control. When confronted with human experiences of a puzzling and indeed mystifying nature we cannot but take recourse to analysis so that we shall be able to disperse our puzzlement or mystification by successfully fragmenting the opaque totality of an experience. Our conditioned response to uncertainty in the face of obscure totalities is that we analyse them. The response is reinforced by the reward of mastery in terms of a self-assurance felt when we proceed into the light cast by the next lamp-post. While entering into its glare we do not fully perceive the darkness beyond and for a while the reward of illumination is therefore great. Now from time to time the notoriously obscurantist complaint is made that, though the explainers of human experience may temporarily dispel mystification and displace metaphysical notions, through their analysis of total and personal experiences they also bring about a disintegration of these experiences (Mannheim, 1946, p. 79). The pertinence of this to the business of psychologists is obvious. In a psychological science inquiry aims at discovering the minutest part of the machinery of experience, for it is assumed in terms of the categories of scientific thinking that understanding of the whole is contingent on the disclosure of parts. Attention to detail is a matter of scientific scrupulousness and pausing to stare at a total picture will be regarded as an inquiry-stopping excuse, a self-deceiving act, or, at best, an aesthetic and non-scientific indulgence. All the same, so far as psychology is analytical and anatomical, so far as it is objective and quantitative, in short, so far as it is rigorously scientific, it is irrevocably landed with the job of examining the function of synthesis in human experience, the function of totalities and of undivided images. It would be less than good psychology to assume that the naïve and spontaneous experience of love will remain unimpaired by analysis and self-consciousness and that it will therefore need no protection against the disruption of this absorbingly total experience.

The important thing to remember, and this is the corner-stone of my hypothesis, is that while the vitalistic psychological teaching of psychoanalysis and of all its derivatives has been, by definition, *analytical*, its moral teaching has *not* been analytical; its ultimate categories of libido, Eros, transference, counter-transference, sublimation, and identification have preserved total, non-fragmental images of *personal* functioning and thereby underpinned and perpetuated traditional moral confidence in a humanistic and noble conception of human love. Meanwhile, the other psychology, which based itself more conscientiously and consistently on physiology or on the simple mechanical notions of learning, has made such a mutual accommodation with traditional moral images of love impossible.

PSYCHOANALYTIC PSYCHOLOGY AND THE GROWTH OF LOVE

To establish some semblance of credibility, I should now like to document the first half of my hypothesis, namely the part that alleges that psychoanalytic psychology explicitly retained the notion of an unanalysable proclivity and need to love and to be loved, and indeed frequently and openly abandoned the claim that this asset of humanity could ever be turned into the alleged small change of physiology or mechanics.

Some most convincing illustrations of this retreat from a scientific position are to be found in the pages of the leading official paper of psychoanalysis, *The International Journal of Psycho-Analysis*. W. R. D. Fairbairn writes there (1958):

'No disparagement of the scientific aspect of psycho-analysis, any more than that of general medicine, is implied in the contention that concern over the scientific aspect of a therapeutic method can be carried too far. For if this concern is too exclusive, the human factor in the therapeutic situation (as represented by individuality, the personal value and the needs of the patient), is only too liable to be sacrificed to the method, which thus comes to assume greater importance than the aims which it is intended to serve.'

It is not only that the aims are *par excellence* moral and non-scientific, but that the 'human factor' – whatever that may mean psychoanalytically – is extraneous and is not to be dissolved in the technicalities of method. Or, to take another testimony from the pages of the same journal:

'. . . the analyst may become a scientific observer to the extent to which he is able to observe objectively the patient and himself in interaction. The interaction itself, however, cannot be adequately represented by the model of scientific neutrality' (Loewald, 1960).

The dissent from the positivistic principles of science is entirely unambiguous. The analyst must use himself as an instrument of therapy and enter into a 'communion' (*sic!*) with his patient, writes another analyst (Foulkes, 1961). Dr L. J. Saul, a training analyst, and Niels Nielson, his colleague – to mention only two, and there are many others – speak of the 'soul' and of the 'spiritual' (Saul, 1958; Nielson, 1960) as if these were recognized parts of Freud's famous 'anatomy' of the mental personality. From Otto Rank (1958, p. 63) to Erich Fromm (1957), mystical and inspirational writing on the spiritual nature and centrality of human love has totally counterbalanced the analytic, reductive, and therefore morally suspect influences of clinical and psychoanalytic ideas.

The 'spiritual' and the 'soul' are eschatologically loaded terms that are brought into the proceedings of a psychoanalytic theory rather as emigré royal dukes are invited to serve on the boards of directors of dubious business organizations. These noble qualities that the analyst is invited to cultivate cannot be accounted for in terms of psychoanalytic theory. If the realities to which these terms of pathos and of ancient reverence relate are mere defences, rationalizations, or projective systems, why hide behind the respectability of these terms? I believe that the authors' solemnity is not a sign of hypocrisy but an unconscious admission by them that they have abandoned their positivistic categories of thinking.

In addition to the reverent use of terms, such as 'soul', 'spiritual', 'communion', and the like, the prescriptions to the practising analyst consistently follow up the implications of these theological gestures. For example, Ruth Strauss in her paper on 'Countertransference' (1960) notes that some patients 'need to have the experience of *merging with the analyst* in order to relieve the pain of separation and thus grow strong enough to give up those fantasies and defences which cut them off from reality' (italics mine). Here, in the context of an applied science, the concept of 'merging' is used as a total unanalysable concept. It describes the therapist's complementary function in a relationship. This relationship is made to look like the *unio mystica* of mother and child, or, for that matter, of man and his god. Similarly, D. W. Winnicott holds (1958, p. 279) that regressed and psychotic patients whose problems are pre-Oedipal in origin and who crave *mothering* above all must be '. . . managed and not analysed'. Guntrip very rightly points out that as the roots of the psychoneuroses always reach back to pre-Oedipal soil, so

> 'the sharp line of demarcation Winnicott draws between management for the psychotic and psycho-analysis for the psychoneurotic breaks down. The position that seems to be emerging is that at all stages psychotherapy has to be an appropriate mixture of mothering (management) and analysis (giving insight). The deeper the level on which treatment has to operate, the greater the patient's need for the mothering he failed to obtain' (Guntrip, 1961, p. 413).

Ontogenetically, the deprivation suffered by the patient is a deprivation of the kind of *primal loving*, of absolute and unconditional loving, which might be weakened by analysis. Arnold Eisendorfer, in his paper in *The Psychoanalytical Quarterly*, writes (1959): 'Empathy . . . refers to the capacity for reciprocal identification between the participants in the interview, i.e. an ability to identify.' The serious pursuit of this idea of 'reciprocal identification' in a psychoanalytic journal discloses continuities with an earlier and mystical type of thinking in which the image of reciprocity in a relationship of love is a condition of salvation. Once again we are presented with a total and personal concept of 'relationship' in a professional relationship of concern or compassion. Another psychoanalyst, Heinrich Racker, explains in the same journal (1958):

> 'to understand is to overcome the division into two (patient and therapist) . . . To understand, to unite with another, and hence also to love prove, at root, to be one and the same. Therefore, understanding is equivalent to positive countertransference, *taking this term in its widest sense to mean love and union*' (italics mine).

The significance of these psychoanalytic excursions into mysticism cannot be over-stressed. These are not instances of 'antiparty' diversionism or exceptional cases of error, but rather expressions of a deeply felt conviction which is extraneous to science. Psychoanalytic psychology is adapted to satisfy both of two opposed metaphysical demands: on the one hand, in moods of positivistic rigour we are invited to look upon Eros and Thanatos as labels of mere biophysical processes; on the other, the nebulously total and personal quality of these categories helps them to acquire a spiritual connotation whenever desired, and so it happens that they are often marshalled to underpin certain types of traditional and inspirational writing on conduct and institutional life. Psychologies that originate in psychoanalytical clinical ideas and therapeutic aspirations are often difficult to discriminate from poetic-theological texts such as, for example, those of Martin Buber (1937).

These excerpts could be easily multiplied but my sample will suffice to indicate that the pieties and traditional respect for the notion of 'spirituality' in love are often enough perpetuated by the vitalistic philosophy of psychoanalysis and of its derivatives. In spite of *The future of an illusion* (Freud, 1928), psychoanalytic modes of thought have powerfully come to the aid of Christian spirituality and of traditional moral images. A simplified and popularized casuistry of these modes of thought has been disseminated through the mass media of communication and this not only has continued to be entirely inoffensive to Christian ways of feeling about fellowship, but has actually strengthened these ways by the constant advocacy of tolerance, permissiveness, and turn-the-other-cheek pedagogy and penology. Richard Lapière (1960) seems to me to be mistaken in regarding the moral influence of psychoanalytic psychology as corrupting. Lapière's charge against psychoanalysis is that it is 'a doctrine of social irresponsibility and personal despair'. My illustrations of the psychoanalytic moral climate would seem to make these charges somewhat severe.

LEARNING THEORY AND THE GROWTH OF LOVE

If the alleged progress is real, presumably it must be sustained by man's faith in its occurring at all. It could not unfold in the face of man's scepticism. For this reason, man's interpretation of his own experience – his psychological interpretation of his role in the social process – is an important determinant of the reality of progress. Our psychological interpretations may help or prejudge the naïve and spontaneous practice of love and compassion. I have been trying to show that the so-called vitalistic-psychoanalytical mode of thought has been an ally of love in its alleged growth among men. Let me now turn to another type of psychological inquiry which has been going on parallel with – though not entirely unmindful of – psychoanalytical and similar thinking. Not unlike vitalistic psychology, this second mainstream of contemporary psychology has had many names and many constituent rivulets. On the whole, these originate partly from the hinterland of physiology and mechanics, and nowadays much of this second stream passes between the banks of so-called learning theories. There are perhaps fewer swamps and misty turnings along this tributary to our present pool of psychological knowledge than there are along the other stream, though at times it is suggested that this tributary is more navigable for vessels conveying animals. To depart from the over-stretched metaphor: the second part of my hypothesis is that the mechanistic psychology of the twentieth century has a conceptual system and a manner of formulating the paradigm experiences of man which may exert an influence on the progression of social changes, presumably representing a kind of 'progress in love and compassion', radically different from what previous vitalistic psychologies have done in this respect.

I propose to illustrate the purport of this apprehensive thesis from recent psychological literature.

Writing about 'Love in infant monkeys', H. F. Harlow (1959) presents his, by now, famous tale of motherless rhesus monkeys, and concludes: '. . . there appears to be no reason why we cannot at some future time investigate the fundamental neurophysiological and biochemical variables underlying affection and love'. Clearly there is a promise here – also implied in psychoanalysis but entirely forgotten there – of penetrating into the very structure and molecular make-up of the response-system called 'love', which, I am sure it will be agreed, is a human experience of some moment. There are no vague notions of spirituality in this psychology or allusions to 'communion' or 'union'; the total or molar and personal experience is equated with the sum of its parts, which are discoverable and shall be discovered. The analytic dismemberment of experience is a necessary and worthy enterprise which the retention of total and personalistic imagery would only obstruct. There is no confluence here between a conveniently ambiguous psychological entelechy, such as, for example, the 'libido', capable of metamorphosing into a kind of

o

fervent affirmation or love, on the one hand, and into the ancient spiritual entelechies on the other. The Harlows in another paper speak of an 'affectional system' which, as systems usually do, consists of identifiable parts or elements. They retain the total concept of 'system' without implying that there might be something specific about a system that a sum or even organization of the parts does not possess. They write: 'It seems possible – even likely – that the infant-mother affectional system is dispensable whereas the infant-infant system is the *sine qua non* for later adjustment in all spheres of monkey life' (Harlow & Harlow, 1962). I shall not digress here to consider the soundness or otherwise of the hypothesis offered here about the importance of inter-stimulation between members of the same litter and about the significance of this to man. Instead, I should like to comment on the analytic etiquette of the scientist which prevails upon him to use inverted euphemisms, such as the notion of an 'affectional system', when meaning 'love'. The thesis is clearly this: love is an analysable response-system consisting of parts which in themselves are not love but certain specifiable mechanical events (items of sensory stimulation). The doctrine is not new, but its direct implications for the policy sciences, for the planning and administration of welfare policies, and thus necessarily for the issue of progress in human sympathy, seem to be new. Before I state this issue, however, let me consider, for example, how another psychologist, Lawrence Casler, proceeds from the baseline of this doctrine to a most suggestive challenge which could hardly be ignored by the ideologists of progress. He writes (1961):

'If institutionalization were to become an acceptable, commonplace means of child rearing rather than serving chiefly as a last resort, what gains would accrue to women freed of the necessity of staying at home during the early months of the child's life? If child rearing – regarded by many as the ultimate justification for marriage in twentieth century western society – is put entirely in the hands of professionals, what predictions could be made about the fate of marriage itself?'

And, indeed, what predictions could be made about the fate of human sociability, sympathy, and love? Casler follows the theory recently formulated that when infants are said to have been deprived of maternal love, they have not in fact been deprived of more than the sum total of specifiable sensory stimulations. Casler concludes that one day these may be quantified, pre-packaged, and administered by appropriately trained personnel entirely supplanting and displacing the nursing functions of natural motherhood. Is this a fantasy of an oral-sadistic child or a prediction about the development in psychology's influence on future human relations? Whichever it is, clearly the sentiments elicited by it and those elicited by John Bowlby's ideas on *Maternal care and the growth of love* (1951) profoundly differ.

While to anticipate the superannuation of all human mother-hood may be somewhat premature, an examination of the social impact of this kind of psychologizing is less so. It seems to me that the psychologist would be less of a psychologist if in his sanguine analytical quest he would ignore the consequences of dispensing with a personalistic and total imagery altogether. So long as the large-scale influencing of public opinion, of nursery practices, of institutional arrangements and procedures in health, education, and welfare, is guided by traditional ethical consider-ations or, as it has been to some extent during this century, by a psychoanalytic theoretical system with its moralistic and person-alistic concepts of libido, adjustment, counter-transference, and the like, an atomistic account of social concern and behaviour, discussed in the pages of scientific journals and books only, is not going to lead to radical changes in our experience of loving. But if, in an age in which the channels of information from psycho-logical expert to public have been vastly extended and consoli-dated, we begin to reinterpret the experience of tenderness in the manner of the Harlows' observations, for example, and to disseminate the information and its logical consequences in the manner of Casler's suggestions, then we psychologists are landed with a new and momentous assignment which we cannot shirk: we shall be obliged to investigate the psychological consequences of disseminating psychological theory and interpretation of modal affectional behaviour *on* the modal affectional behaviour so interpreted. Naturally one might argue that a dissolution of the molar and personalistic images of love occurred often, before and since the time of Pavlov, yet this has not impaired the spiritual imagery or the popular romanticization of love, or cooled the sentimental potentials and affectional ardours of people. The psychophysiological interpreters of love have consequently assumed that a naïve and spontaneous affectionateness can coexist and flourish side by side with an exclusively neurophysiological mirror-image of it. Or at least they seem to think that whatever influence they may exert with their version of this paradigm of humanity will make no more mark on man's morality than the previous versions have made, or, for that matter, social science has ever made. I know many psychologists whose theories of love leave the warmth and compassion of their human relationships unaffected. I suppose these psychologists deserve our admiration for the extraordinary skill with which they demonstrate the irrelevance of their thinking to their existence. We may, of course, say that there is plenty of time to look at the future vicissitudes of love after we have learnt a great deal more about its molecular causes and nature.

I feel that we would be complacent to go along with this. The sociopsychological influence of psychological interpretation has considerably grown since the times of the early behaviourists. Today, the casuistry of mostly psychoanalytically inspired mental hygiene is published in the magazine and paperback press, and its psychological prescriptions have become important elements in our social control. Meanwhile the Pavlovian mode of thought too begins to make its overtures to wider audiences:

> 'The Majima Manufacturing Company of Tokio has begun marketing an article called "mother heart" – a breast-shaped device that gives off the sound of heartbeats. It is supposed to put crying babies to sleep' (news item).

Spare parts for rejecting mothers are now available and soon enough the entire assembled article may turn up in our mail-order catalogues. Though this may be a pointer to the future, for the time being there are few signs of a new casuistry begotten by popularized learning theory to influence private conduct. There are as yet few signs of a synthetic love concept actually exerting a moral influence either on parental solicitousness or on the professional dedication of workers in the fields of health and education. 'Love', 'compassion', and 'fellowship' still carry the accumulated reverence of past ages and the complex notions still act as powerful stimuli to socially necessary performances. The new categories, such as, for example, 'sensory stimulation', are not yet used widely in child guidance clinics or in the planning and administration of children's homes. But the first steps have been taken and behavioural scientists are energetically advocating the application of learning theory premises to psychotherapy.

Once again, to illuminate these generalities, I should like to give an example of the context from which my concerns spring. In the recently published *Behaviour therapy and the neuroses*, under the editorship of H. J. Eysenck, there is an abundance of suitable illustration for what I have in mind. If I single out one paragraph, it is entirely because of limitations of space and not for want of suitable passages. A. A. Lazarus reports on the case of a nine-year-old girl whose mother

> '. . . stated that she had read an article which stressed that one should refrain from giving a nine-year-old child any overt demonstrations of love and affection (such as hugging or kissing the child), since these practices supposedly hindered the development of "personality and maturity". The therapist vehemently condemned this contention and provided *"handling instructions"*, which emphasized the necessity for deliberate and overt love and warmth' (Lazarus, 1960, p. 117, italics mine).

If the mode of thought of this psychotherapy is that it advocates 'handling instructions' when in fact it aims at an advocacy of love, we may find that a piecemeal obeisance to it will elicit 'handling' and not 'love'. Whether there are 'do-it-yourself-kits' of loving behaviour or not is a psychological question, but the paradoxical thing is that even a truthful affirmative answer to the question might jeopardize the spontaneous appearance of loving behaviour. Truth may well become self-stultifying by being made known. It is, to say the least, open to doubt that a literal execution of pre-scribed motions, prescribed 'handling', will induce a satisfactory change in unloving mothers or in hurried and harassed institutional staff. It is subject to future sociopsychological inquiry whether the dissemination of this kind of psychological advice via the mass media of communications will not in fact produce a self-stultifying moral climate in which the progress of the regimen of love in human relations might be halted.

One of the most articulate critics of vitalistic psychology, Lady Wootton, provides me with a suitable concluding testimony. Having repudiated the psychoanalytical interpretations of the

concept of maternal deprivation, interpretations mostly associated
with the name of John Bowlby (1951), she concludes:

> 'Up to the present . . . research into the effects of maternal
> deprivation is to be valued chiefly for its incidental exposure of
> the prevalence of deplorable patterns of institutional upbring-
> ing, and of the crass indifference of certain hospitals to childish
> sensitivities. Without doubt this research has already had
> excellent practical effects in stimulating many of the authorities
> responsible for children's homes and hospitals to change their
> ways for the better' (Wootton, 1959, p. 156).

Here we have an entirely unsolicited testimonial from a social
scientist whose 'tough-minded' intellectual rigour would allow
support only to a mechanistic kind of psychology. It says: the
vitalistic theory in question offers us unproven hypotheses but its
moral influence in some areas has been to further progress in the
reduction of 'crass indifference' and, therefore, in the growth of
love. Could we, either opponents or friends of the mechanistic
and learning theories, come to a similar conclusion in respect of
the moral influence of a mechanistic psychology?

If the act of tenderness can be resolved into its mechanical
parts, then it should be possible to reassemble those parts into an
act of tenderness. Could this tenderness have developed fully
without a naïve belief – at least a suspicion or hope – that the
act of tenderness was a total, indivisible, and personal act? The
question is primarily not whether the mechanistic account of love
is true but whether we can continue to progress in love when
everybody thinks it true.

REFERENCES

BOWLBY, J. (1951). *Maternal care and mental health*. World Health
    Organization Technical Monograph Series, No. 2. Geneva.
    Also in abridged version, *Child care and the growth of love*.
    Harmondsworth: Penguin Books, 1953.
BUBER, M. (1937). *I and Thou*. Edinburgh: T. & T. Clark.
CASLER, L. (1961). Maternal deprivation: a critical review of the
    literature. *Monograph of the Society for Research in Child
    Development*, No. 80, Vol. 26, No. 2.

EDER, M. D. (1962). The myth of progress. *Brit. J. med. Psychol.* **35**, 81–9.

EISENDORFER, A. (1959). The selection of candidates applying for psychoanalytic training. *Psychoanal. Quart.* **28**, 374–378.

FAIRBAIRN, W. R. D. (1958). On the nature and aims of psychoanalytic treatment. *Int. J. Psycho-Anal.* **39**, 374–85.

FOULKES, S. H. (1961). Psychotherapy. *Brit. J. med. Psychol.* **35**, 91–102.

FREUD, S. (1928). *The future of an illusion.* Standard Edition Vol. XXI. London: Hogarth.

FROMM, E. (1957). *The art of loving.* London: Allen & Unwin.

GINSBERG, M. (1961). *Evolution and progress.* London: Heinemann.

GUNTRIP, H. (1961). *Personality structure and human interaction.* London: Hogarth.

HALMOS, P. (1957). *Towards a measure of man.* International Library of Sociology. London: Routledge & Kegan Paul.

HARLOW, H. F. (1959). Love in infant monkeys. *Sci. Amer.* June, 68–74.

—— & HARLOW, M. K. (1962). Social deprivation in monkeys. *Sci. Amer.* November, 137–46.

LAPIÈRE, R. (1960). *The Freudian ethic.* London: Allen & Unwin.

LAZARUS, A. A. (1960). The elimination of children's phobias by deconditioning. In H. J. Eysenck (ed.), *Behaviour therapy and the neuroses.* New York: Pergamon Press.

LOEWALD, H. W. (1960). On the therapeutic action of psychoanalysis. *Int. J. Psycho-Anal.* **41**, 16–33.

MANNHEIM, K. (1946). *Ideology and Utopia.* London: Routledge & Kegan Paul.

NIELSON, N. (1960). Value judgments in psycho-analysis. *Int. J. Psycho-Anal.* **41**, 425–9.

RACKER, H. (1958). Psychoanalytic technique and the analyst's unconscious masochism. *Psychoanal. Quart.* **27**, 555–62.

RANK, O. (1958). *Beyond psychology.* New York: Dover.

SAUL, L. J. (1958). *Technic and practice of psychoanalysis.* Philadelphia: Lippincott.

STRAUSS, RUTH (1960). Counter-transference. *Brit. J. med. Psychol.* **33**, 23–7.

WINNICOTT, D. W. (1958). *Collected papers: through paediatrics to psycho-analysis.* London: Tavistock Publications.

WOOTTON, B. (1959). *Social science and social pathology.* London: Allen & Unwin.

Part IV: Conclusions

10 Summary and Conclusions

S. H. FOULKES

Let us look back now on the contributions by the various authors and comment upon them with a view to bringing out their significance for our issue and to seeing what conclusions their evidence will support.

I would ask the reader to bear in mind in following this review that I am speaking from the standpoint of group analysis as it has been developed from my own experience in group-analytic psychotherapy and its applications to the therapeutic community, to teaching, and to training. If this method, orientation, and attitude are relevant to the kinds of problem with which we are concerned in this volume, I am bound to take this as my point of departure. Indeed, the approach to the problem of the Section as I found it and as has been described in the Introductory was deliberately chosen as a demonstration of group-analytic principles in action. The existing controversy within the Section was made the basis of the Section's transactions during the year of my Chairmanship.

Dr Hare's contribution has been included especially as an authoritative statement of the opposite view of social psychiatry to that otherwise presented in this book. Dr Hare wisely reminds us of the dangers of being over-preoccupied with terminology and, by pointing out the parallels between social psychiatry and social medicine, warns us against dogmatism in considering a field as complex as this. Furthermore, in emphasizing that the social psychiatrist is concerned with the three areas of treatment, research, and prevention, he shows that clear distinctions are probably premature in this complex field, in that most psychotherapists will claim the same trio of concerns.

Let us turn to the joint paper by Professor Meyer Fortes and Dr Doris Mayer. Professor Fortes, who is Professor of Anthropology at Cambridge, revisited the Tallensi tribe whom he had

studied intimately thirty years earlier. Their region in the north
of Ghana presents a striking contrast with the south of that
country, an industrial area much influenced by contact with the
Western world.

Professor Fortes was struck by the fact that thirty years ago
there had been only one case of madness and two somewhat
queer people, one perhaps a psychotic, the other more likely a
defective, among the population he met. Now there were thirteen
Tallensi and seven of the neighbouring Gorensi who were
undoubtedly psychotic. After other explanations had been considered and rejected, it seemed certain that this difference had to
do with the social contact with the south of Ghana. All of the
psychoses were acquired by these people when they were living
in the south or very shortly after they returned from there.

Dr Doris Mayer, who is a psychiatrist, examined these cases
carefully. She ruled out any borderline or doubtful cases. She
found that symptoms corresponded more or less to those known in
Western psychiatry. However, her patients were more willing to talk
than were the American patients to whom she was accustomed,
since among the Tallensi no stigma was attached to hallucinations.
A significant difference was that *kindly* voices, encouraging voices,
were predominant. Dr Mayer suggested that this may be associated with the very gradual way in which children in this tribe go
through their transitional stages of childhood, including weaning.
There were clearly precipitating upsetting events which triggered
off the psychotic breakdowns. Another interesting observation
was that these patients responded extremely well to doses of
medicine that were quite inadequate in quantity to have any
pharmacological effect.

These psychotic breakdowns were undoubtedly precipitated by
stress, in that the social, economic, and cultural horizons had
expanded enormously in these thirty years. National and political
movements and propaganda have changed the traditional value
system. The Tallensi are at a critical point of transition and in a
state of far-reaching change. There is incompatibility between
the still stable traditional internal organization of the family and
the external social, economic, and ideological sphere. (We are
reminded here of the pioneer work of one of Professor Fortes's
teachers, Professor C. G. Seligman, who so early and so clearly
stressed the cross-cultural aspects of psychosis, culture-bound

forms of pathological states such as delusions and paranoid states.)

I should like at this point to contrast these observations with a statement in *Clinical psychiatry* by Mayer-Gross, Slater, and Roth (1954). It is as follows:

'Now if social factors in causation were known to influence the incidence and distribution of psychotic disorders they would be of the utmost importance for social psychiatry.'

They go on to say that these facts have not yet been established, that if they were they would have a bearing on the work of the clinician, but

'in the meantime the psychiatric clinician will have to be guided by the information on which he can rely, that which he himself has gathered from the study of individual patients. While he will maintain an interest in sociology as a field of research which impinges on society he will rate the sociological causes of illness at what seems to him the importance they deserve. In the psychoses they will be low on the list, in the neuroses generally higher.'

The contribution by Professor Fortes and Dr Mayer is in itself a study of the manifestations of change in a society which is in the process of changing.

There is clear evidence here that psychoses of a schizophrenic type were observed during the anthropologist's second visit, whereas only one or two cases had been observed thirty years before. It seems also beyond reasonable doubt that the occurrence of these psychoses had to do with the social and cultural changes in the lives of the population. The last point is demonstrated with the exactitude almost of an experiment. Although Professor Fortes did not in this case visit the country with the intention of making a specific study of this problem and precise statistical material is therefore not available, nevertheless his intimate acquaintance with every single family in the community, together with the fact that he was struck by the sudden emergence of psychotic illness which had been practically absent previously, must give validity to his observation.

On the psychiatric side, Dr Mayer has clearly confirmed the diagnoses. Her remarks on the similarities as well as the differences between psychotic illnesses in Northern Ghana and in Europe or the United States are of high interest.

We come now to studies from Britain, from school, from industry, and from hospital.

In his contribution from the field of education, Mr Lyward reported on his lifelong experience and how this led him from teaching to therapy. The most important point is that he came to therapeutic work largely as the result of many years' exploration of how best to teach subjects. The sentence 'These are people – we are all people together in a room – that is the most important fact about this situation' is enormously significant. Stress on the child as a whole person and on the need for understanding emotional problems and, above all, listening to them should be familiar to any psychotherapist or social psychiatrist, and he speaks significantly of the group life. He underlines the importance of maintaining 'group life at depth' and adds 'that depth is vital to its members'. This might well be a direct message to the Section in its current situation.

The emphasis on the value of listening is underlined in the all-too-short contribution from Professor Revans. The strength of the relation between level of work-satisfaction and 'good listening' or 'bad listening' on the part of management is surely impressive. His study also underlines the importance of the group. He speaks of the opposition to change so well known to us in psychotherapy as resistance. He describes a method of quantifying attitudes to change, which should stimulate thought for those engaged in the practice of psychiatry where the quantification of the outcome of treatment is notoriously difficult. His phrase 'nobody wants to learn until he admits his need to do so' is also significant.

Miss Menzies reports an approach to disturbance at a hospital which may serve as a perfect example of social psychiatry in action, using the term 'social psychiatry' as understood in this volume. Indeed, the most significant fact of her study is perhaps that she was consulted as a psychotherapist. She describes her research method as sociotherapy and stresses that the main task is a therapeutic one, the research findings resulting in a secondary way. This approach will be familiar to those psychiatrists who maintain that there is no diagnosis without treatment. A study of a community conducted in this manner provides access to aspects of the situation which would be totally concealed in more conventional researches.

It need hardly be said that the principles applied by Miss Menzies are close to those of group analysis. In fact she makes these principles very clear, both in the description of the method and in the underlying attitude. In stating that she does clinical research, research in relation to an actual problem which causes distress, she shows the particular advantages as well as the difficulties of such research. She is right in saying that the nature of communication changes, that it goes deeper, that its freedom increases, that one gains access to levels which otherwise are not articulated or manifest in any way. Her attitude is very much that of the analyst in that she proceeds from the presenting problem or symptom to the underlying real trouble and in that she prefers a relatively unstructured situation. She mentions the difficulty of providing data which can be measured and used statistically under such conditions. Miss Menzies offers a hypothesis about the defensive function of some organizational systems against anxiety which she compares with the corresponding psychic defences in the individual patient. I want to stress particularly Miss Menzies's work as an example of clinical or action research, the most appropriate way, in my opinion, of research in social psychiatry.

Research, diagnosis, and therapy are here interconnected. Miss Menzies quite clearly directs her therapy to the group-as-a-whole. In the strictly therapeutic group, the group-as-a-whole is in our view considered as the all-embracing context of all ongoing dynamics, though the individual patient is more in the centre of therapy than is the case when the 'patient' is an organization or institution. When the group-as-a-whole takes an active part in the process of therapy it follows that it is aware of the disturbance and asking for assistance.

We come now to three more theoretical contributions by Elias, Chance, and Halmos.

Professor Norbert Elias as a sociologist has long recognized that so-called precise studies based on objective measurements alone are quite misleading and insufficient. He maintains that it is necessary for the sociologist to cooperate with the psychoanalyst and, perhaps in particular, with the group analyst.

Dr Elias sees psychiatry and sociology as two distinct disciplines and social psychiatry as an interdisciplinary field – a borderland.

He examines the desirable rapprochement and its problems from an interactional point of view. He sees as essential an understanding on two levels at the same time, namely the individual and the group level. He finds a general theoretical significance in such a two-level approach beyond that in psychotherapy.

It could be said, moreover, that in an approach such as that adopted by Miss Menzies or in group analysis there is in fact an *integration* of these two levels. In actual observation they can hardly be kept apart. The manners and customs of his society are built centrally into the individual and are not external. Although this integration has been achieved for a considerable time in clinical practice, it is much more difficult to give a theoretical account of the process. It is made more difficult by the fact that all our concepts are charged with meaning which carries with it this dichotomy, 'individual versus group', as a heritage from our particular individual upbringing and tradition. Eventually I found most useful the concept of a total interactional dynamic network. The forces and processes transact inside this total network. They are not merely interpersonal but transpersonal, that is to say they penetrate through and pass through the individuals who form in a sense nodal points in a total interacting system (Foulkes, 1964).

Dr Elias made a plea for cooperation, but he also envisages integration, and acknowledges that 'great steps have already been made in this kind of vision, particularly in the group-analytic approach'. As if in response to our segregationalists, Elias states in *The established and the outsiders* (Elias & Scotson, 1965):

> 'Models of configurations of social patterns or structures can be no less precise and reliable than the results of quantitative measurement of isolated factors or variables. What they lack is a deceptive finality of inferences based on quantitative analysis alone which is often mistaken for precision.'

Later on, he states:

> 'Other aspects of the inquiry too indicated that in this social context inferences from statistical analysis of interviews alone were of limited value without the knowledge acquired by means of a systematic inquiry by a trained participant observer.'

Dr Chance, a biologist, believes that an exact science of human behaviour can be established on the basis of ethology. His contribution is of interest on methodological grounds as well as those of theory. He links up with Dr Elias and myself in stressing how conventional terms colour and prejudice observations. There is also an important step in the direction of putting social behaviour and the group into the centre of reference. Dr Chance speaks of 'patterns of events without experimental interference'. His illustrations from a description of sub-human primate social behaviour are fascinating and his concluding paragraphs are particularly pertinent. His emphasis on the need for acceptance of change whether in the individual or in the group and on the forces which inhibit or facilitate change might have come from a psychotherapist.

Professor Halmos stressed the influence of psychological theories on society. He showed how certain doctrines tended to influence social behaviour quite apart from their inherent truth or otherwise. He illustrated this particularly in connection with psychoanalysis, on the one side, and the new brand of behaviourism in psychology, on the other.

Dr Halmos linked the doctrine of progress and the growth of love with certain developments in psychotherapy and psychoanalysis. He appears to me to neglect in this the importance of aggressive and destructive tendencies. He thinks that psychoanalysis retreats from a scientific position as regards the ethical values. He speaks of theological gestures, of mythical and inspirational writing. He quotes in this connection as an example the use of the term 'communion' with the patient. As used by myself, this was meant to express the fact that on that level no active process of communication is necessary because the mind of the therapist and that of the patient are in complete unison and in contact with each other. No mythical, mystical, or quasi-religious notions are involved. I might refer to Kellman (1959), who uses the term 'communing' perhaps in a similar sense. The prototype is that of the early mother-child relationship which has its correspondence in the transference situation (see Rof Carballo, 1960). If there is some justification for the shift which Professor Halmos seems to see in psychoanalysis it would seem to me to lie in the following:

1. Psychoanalysis has penetrated into the personality in greater depth partly through a refinement of the structural approach

(a dynamic and interactional view of ego, superego, and id, particularly in their unconscious aspects) and partly through the closer study of early childhood influences (particularly by Melanie Klein, 1932). This has led to more emphasis being put on the pre-oedipal stages and on very early child-mother relationships.

2. There is more emphasis on the thorough analysis of the ongoing transference situation, sometimes referred to as the 'here and now', by contrast to the reductive analysis which tended to base the investigation as thoroughly as possible on the re-experience, remembrance, and reconstruction of child-hood events. This development was foreshadowed by Ferenczi and Rank in 1924 (Ferenczi & Rank, 1924).

3. There is perhaps a shift from the importance allotted to insight, even of an intellectual kind, towards that of a working-through, an experiencing under changed conditions and with new understanding. It has, of course, always been understood that insight without emotional experience is of very limited value. Another way of formulating these developments would be to speak of a tendency in the direction of a more existential, experiential approach as it has long been represented in psycho-analytic circles by Binswanger (1963).

Of course, insight was always understood in psychoanalysis not as predominantly intellectual insight but as emotional insight; yet looking back on the first few decades of psychoanalytic development one discerns that relatively greater importance was attached to more or less intellectual insight.

I myself am with Professor Halmos in placing special value on the scientific nature of the analytical investigation and attitude; but, as has been explained in different parts of the present volume, the intervention of the examiner, therapist, or observer must be taken into account so that the scientific process itself appears in a different light from that in which it would have appeared to Freud in the early part of the century. I believe that observations in psychoanalysis and group analysis are of particular value in assessing the therapeutic processes and their theoretical clarifi-cation.

Be that as it may, the particular value of Professor Halmos's contribution, apart from its thought-provoking nature, lies in the fact that he dynamically examines the interaction between psychological theories and social behaviour in our own society.

Is it too much to hope that the Section might consider it one of its future tasks to act not only as a forum for such reports – danger signals for the health of the community as they are – but as consultants if necessary, to intervene and to institute further research? Symposia could be organized of groups of participants representing different factions concerning hospitals, industry, education, law, and so on.

We can claim that the evidence confirms all that we set out to prove. The problems met at the present time by quite independent observers, distinguished experts in their own fields of work, have much in common. So have the methods developed as an approach to these problems for investigation and amelioration, as well as the attitudes which have been found to be most useful.

The problems in their central core are psychiatric ones, more specifically they are psychotherapeutic challenges. Not only are they in their nature inseparable from those for which psychiatrists are traditionally consulted but also they present themselves clearly as 'dis-eases' expressed by symptoms asking for relief or cure. The therapeutic model suggests itself as the most relevant and adequate. An approach has to include psychoanalytical insights such as the power of the emotions, of unconscious meaning, the nature of resistances and defences, transferences, built-in values and attitudes, and so forth. The evidence supports in particular the basic postulates of group analysis.

This book is an account of a year's work within the Psychotherapy and Social Psychiatry Section of the Royal Medico-Psychological Association. The address from the Chair traditionally takes place at the end of the term. I shall end this review by putting forward a few points which were formulated in my Chairman's address as they seem to me to have emerged from the year's work.

1. A field for social psychiatry exists which is of central importance for psychiatry and psychotherapy as regards research and practice.

2. Problems arising in various fields, for instance, anthropology,

education, industry, administration, are similar and interrelated. They are essentially problems in social psychology and psychiatry.

3. Social and cultural factors determine the individual's inner structure decisively. Syndromes and diseases, their very existence and the form they take, cannot be understood outside their sociocultural context, neither in their nature nor as regards their cure.

4. The study of small groups, in particular of an analytical kind, has proved a good instrument for practice and research in this social field.

5. A scientific approach in ongoing life is possible. Clinical research, therapeutic research, action research, also in the light of ongoing problems in society, can be valid and precise.

6. The concept of scientific detachment is outdated. It is pseudo-scientific. The hallmark of a scientific attitude is respect for and accordance with the realities of any given situation ascertained with a minimum of prejudice.

7. We must get away from a false impartiality in favour of a conscious participation in the service of humanity. Analysis of the values which we respect or intend to support, and of which we are often unaware, must precede action, which can then take the form of an enlightened participation.

I have mentioned the way in which this Section's function can be seen in the light of this evidence and I need not repeat this. In my view, the Section should take up the position which rightly belongs to it – a meeting-ground for the concerns of all disciplines to demonstrate that similar changes are taking place and occupying researchers in all fields of human endeavour at the same time and for the same reason.

Using the conflict in the Psychotherapy and Social Psychiatry Section of the Royal Medico-Psychological Association as a dramatization, group-analytic study has revealed the far-reaching and deep-going conflicts that lay behind it. As to the Section itself, Dr Hare and his colleagues may well find that they can work only in a section of their own or as part of a more general 'scientific section'. I would agree with Dr Hare and with Sir

Aubrey Lewis that it would have been wrong for the Section to become yet another psychotherapeutic society. Members of different analytic schools may feel that they too want sections of their own, which indeed they have in their different societies. They may feel disturbed by sociologists and others who do not share the experience of the thoroughbred psychoanalyst, in particular his access to the 'unconscious'. It seems that what people should do in this situation is to learn – by facing new facts and, if possible, by experiencing and participating.

REFERENCES

BINSWANGER, L. (1963). *Being-in-the-world.* New York: Basic Books.

ELIAS, N. & SCOTSON, J. L. (1965). *The established and the outsiders.* London: Frank Cass.

FERENCZI, S. & RANK, O. (1924). *Entwicklungsziele der Psycho-analyse.* Leipzig/Wien/Zürich: Internationaler Psychoanaly-tischer Verlag.

FOULKES, S. H. (1964). *Therapeutic group analysis.* London: Allen & Unwin.

KELLMANN, A. (1959). Communing and relating. *Amer. J. Psychoanal.* **24.**

KLEIN, M. (1932). *The psycho-analysis of children.* London: Hogarth.

MAYER-GROSS, W., SLATER, E. S. & ROTH, M. (1954). *Clinical psychiatry.* London: Cassell.

ROF CARBALLO, J. (1960). Constitution, transference and co-existence. *Acta psychother.* **8.**